Pole Dance Fitness

Irina Kartaly

POLE DANCE

FITNESS

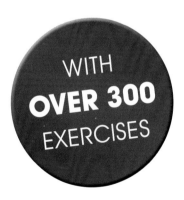

WITH
OVER 300
EXERCISES

Meyer & Meyer Sport

British Library Cataloguing in Publication Data
A catalogue record for this book is available from the British Library

Pole Dance Fitness
Maidenhead: Meyer & Meyer Sport (UK) Ltd., 2018
ISBN 978-1-78255-126-3

4th reprint 2021 of the 1st edition 2018

Aachen, Auckland, Beirut, Dubai, Hägendorf, Hong Kong, Indianapolis, Cairo, Cape Town,
Manila, Maidenhead, New Delhi, Singapore, Sydney, Teheran, Vienna

 Member of the World Sports Publishers' Association (WSPA)

Credits
Design & Layout:
Cover & Interior Design: Annika Naas
Typesetting: www.satzstudio-hilger.de
Cover and Chapter Opener Photos: © Checo13.photography
Exercise Photos: © Gearbox Studios
Editorial:
Managing Editor: Elizabeth Evans
Copyeditor: Anne Rumery
Manufacturing: Print Consult GmbH, Munich, Germany

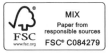

ISBN 978-1-78255-126-3
E-mail: info@m-m-sports.com
www.m-m-sports.com

CONTENTS

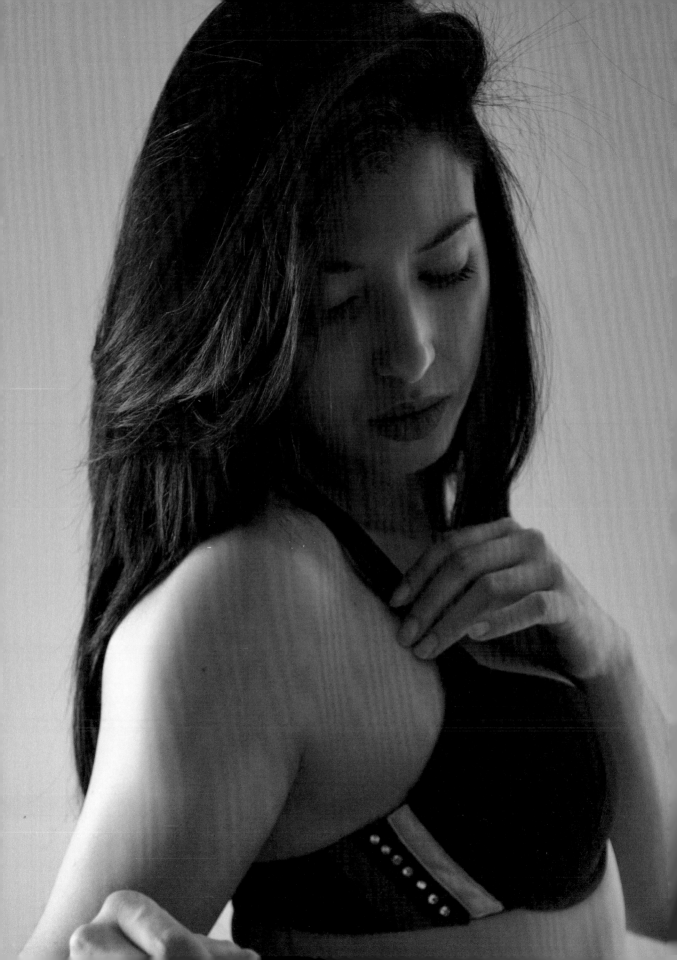

ACKNOWLEDGMENTS

I would like to express my gratitude to those who supported and participated in the creation of this book: Meyer & Meyer Sports for allowing me to take on this project; my talented coach, Iraima Aular, and all pole athletes around the world from whom I have learned so much. Special recognition goes to my consultants, Nour Ezz, Dr. Han Salvedia, Michel Nabil, Mahmoud Zag, and Alexandra Aftanase; the models Germana Viafara and Monica Ochoa for their participation; Checo13.photography; Gearbox Studios; and all of the collaborators for their assistance with and support for this successful work.

Above all, I thank God for making this project possible, and for the guidance and enormous amount of love given. I thank my beloved mother, father, sister, and husband, who have stood by me every step of the way and who have always been my main inspiration.

To my family and country whom I'll always hold dear to my heart: this is for you and to honor you.

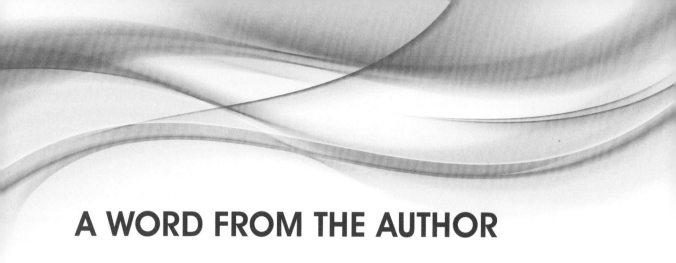

A WORD FROM THE AUTHOR

Pole dance is an athletic discipline performed by men and women of all ages with a wide variety of body structures, physical characteristics, and backgrounds, and at all levels of sports experience or dancing skills. The main objective of this pole dance and fitness book is to serve as a guideline for and to encourage all enthusiasts and instructors who choose to practice this challenging sport.

The popularity of pole dance has grown over the years due to the multiple benefits it provides, including physical, cognitive, psychological, social, and emotional development; improvement of muscle tone, body strength, mobility, flexibility, stamina, kinesthetic awareness, coordination, motor skills, neuromuscular control, and psychological and emotional stress release. It also contributes to self-esteem and self-confidence by simultaneously combining sensuality, grace, a healthier lifestyle, and a fitter body complemented by each person's individual qualities. Progress varies for each performer according to their characteristics, and training frequency, among other influential factors. However, it is important to remember that it takes time for the mind and body to acknowledge and assimilate the new demands of the exercises and movements being performed.

In this pole dance and fitness guide, readers will find specific information with practical descriptions and illustrations to help them understand the most appropriate approach for each exercise, movement, trick, or spin, including detailed exercise sets for workouts and stretching before and after the execution of pole dance tricks. This information is planned to progressively condition and prepare the body for the consequent challenges on the pole through technical notes for each pole figure and spin according to its level of difficulty, unique compositions of pole dance transitions to combine and create different dance and acrobatic routines, and postural exercises to improve body posture and alignment.

There are numerous aspects to consider in the practice of pole dance. As an enthusiast and coach, I highly recommend dedicating special attention to safety measures and the procurement of a certified pole dance instructor's assistance. Remember, this is a high-risk sport in which aerial stunts are performed. The pole dance and fitness guide is in no way meant to be substitute for proper instruction; it is expected to be used as a guideline and a valuable tool for dancers surrounded by a safe environment and in conjunction with personal or group training. Another valuable aspect to be consider is technique and the progressive manner in which the tricks and spins must be performed. Bear in mind that it is not a matter of quantity but quality. Investing more time on a trick's execution improves the performer's skills and ensures further satisfactory results.

The process is continuous and progressive; prepare to marvel at your achievements.

—Irina Kartaly

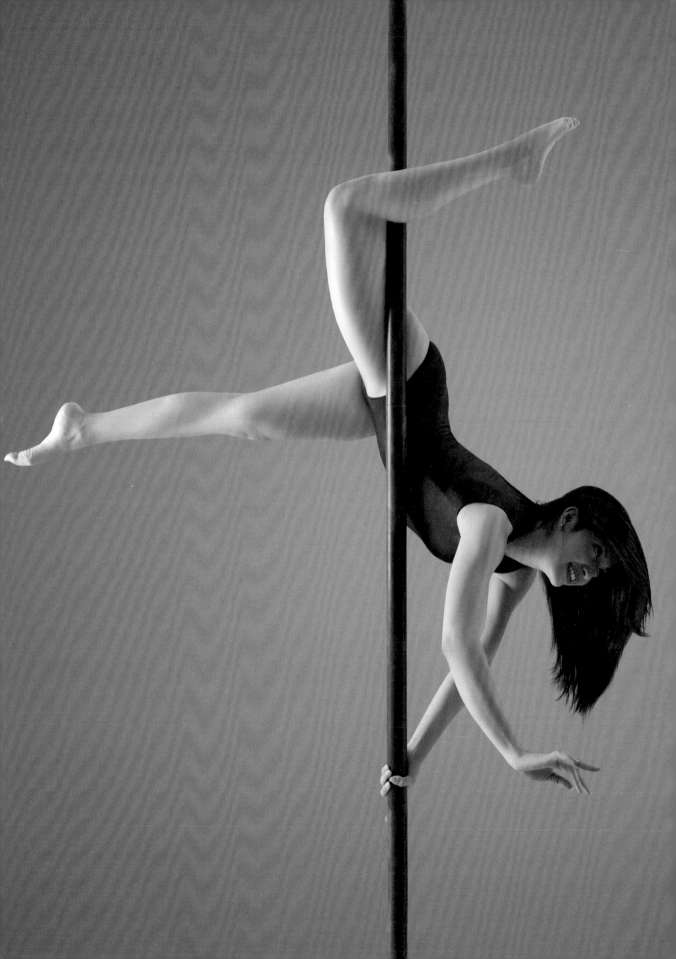

POLE DANCE AND FITNESS:
GENRES, POLES, AND PRODUCTS

Pole dance and fitness is an athletic discipline that combines dance routines, acrobatic stunts, and a vertical pole. Pole dance performance requires significant muscular endurance, coordination, and flexibility for the movements and spins. It can be considered both an aerobic and anaerobic exercise. Upper body, core, and lower body strength, along with proper instruction and continuous training and conditioning are essential to the process.

Over time, pole dance has grown into a discipline and a sport practiced at numerous dance and fitness studios in many countries. Pole athletes can even participate in national, international, amateur, and professional competitions around the world. Considered a leisure activity and a performance art, all performers are motivated by the benefits provided by its practice.

POLE DANCE GENRES

- **Pole fitness:** Concentrates mainly on physical strength and technical aspects for each of the movements and stunts with conditioning-focused exercises.

- **Artistic pole and acrobatics:** Emphasizes dance and expression, and focuses on movement and music, including choreography and acrobatic stunts. Different dance styles might be incorporated in this category according to the performer's preferences.

- **Exotic pole:** Possesses a more sensual approach. The performer usually incorporates high heels to the choreography which stresses movements requiring flexibility, as well as grounded transitional movements, commonly known as floor work.

THE POLES

There is a variety of poles to suit different approaches according to the performer's requirements and purposes. Dance poles can have static or spinning modes, be portable or permanent, can vary in size, height, and thickness, and be made with different coatings or materials.

There are numerous pole manufacturers worldwide which provide high-quality products to ensure a safe performance for pole dance enthusiasts.

Permanent poles are fixed to the ceiling and supported by girders anchored to the ground by brackets. Depending to the pole manufacturer and brand, there are different manners in which to install and fix the pole in a given location. Portable poles are supported by a base or a portable stand and do not need to be attached to the ceiling. These poles are easily dismantled and can be transported to different locations. There are also portable poles which work by pressure, and are designed to be installed and dismantled according to the performer's requirements. Transportation and storage is easy and the extension of the pole can be modified with specific measured pole extensions.

The pole diameters for dance and fitness vary (e.g., 40 mm, 45 mm, and 50 mm) depending on the usage purpose and personal preferences including the challenger's characteristics. The most common classification is for studio or competition use.

The poles may have both spinning and static modes, while others may only provide one or the other. Spinning poles use ball bearings in order to spin, while static poles do not allow rotation or spin, remaining in a fixed position. Each mode provides different advantages and it is highly recommended to practice and perform on both pole modes, to avoid becoming accustomed to one or the other which limits the improvement of skill development, performance, and progress in general.

There is a diversity of pole materials and coatings, each of which have their own different properties and advantages. Poles may be brass, titanium, gold, stainless steel, or chrome. There are also silicon- and powder-coated poles, which provide maximum grip for the user. However, silicon poles require challengers to cover their skin with clothing in order to avoid direct skin contact and any lacerations that may result. Silicon-coated poles are recommended to be used only for certain tricks and performers, since it might not contribute to the challenger's grip-strength development. Usually used in a static mode, powder-coated poles can also provide optimum grip and friction while performing. The brass, titanium, or gold poles increase the performer's grip and are often used by advanced challengers. Stainless steel poles, however, provide a moderate grip in contrast to the others, and are usually used by performers with more sensitive skin. Last but not least, the most popular pole material (and one that is often used by beginner performers) is silver chrome.

PRODUCTS

It is common to apply different products to the pole and on various body parts, such as magnesium, Mighty Grip, Dry Hands, or iTac2. Performers also continuously wipe the pole with isopropyl alcohol (or other products, as advised by the pole's manufacturers) to improve the grip on the pole; it may also depend on the performer's preferences, characteristics, skin type, pole material, and environment. These products are highly recommended for challengers who suffer from hyperhidrosis, but regular application is also inadvisable in order to avoid minimizing strength development on the pole.

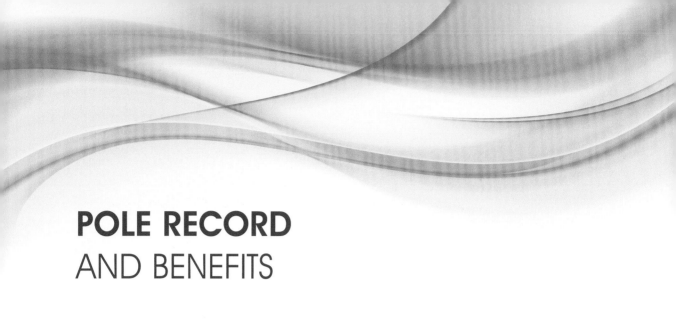

POLE RECORD
AND BENEFITS

Pole dance has grown in popularity over the years in many countries around the world. Its existence dates back to the twelfth century with 9-meter poles used by Chinese circus performers. Full-body outfits and costumes were used to grip the rubber-covered poles. Performances were less fluent and choreographed, and performers mainly executed aerial stunts, flips, jumps, climbs, and contortions, as well as holding suspended positions, usually performed by more than two challengers at once. Nowadays, spectators around the world can appreciate performances of Cirque Du Soleil which is very much influenced by these Chinese circuses.

In India, the traditional Maharashtra performances are over 800 years old, and are still practiced in competitions around the country, using a tapered wooden pole with a base diameter of 55 cm and 35 cm diameter at the top. As in modern day pole dance and fitness, skin exposure was required to provide proper grip to the pole. Although there were pole dance competitions, it was mainly used by wrestlers as a training practice to improve speed and develop coordination, reflexes, and concentration. Because it requires agility and precision, and increases the performer's endurance, strength, flexibility, and stamina, pole dance has proven to be beneficial for other athletic activities.

In the 1920s, during the Great Depression in the United States, travelling fair performers known as the Hoochie Coochie would dance around a tent's support pole, entertaining spectators with fluent hip movements and body exposure. Pole dance is commonly mistaken for an exotic dance form due to its use in adult entertainment establishments, but in reality, this is far from the true essence of pole dance as an athletic discipline. Pole athletes who perform with an exotic approach require as much practice, training, and dedication as those in other pole dance disciplines.

There are pole dance recordings from 1968 in the U.S., and by the 80s, it was popular in Canada, as well. By 1994, the first pole dancing school was created by Fawnia Dietrich, along with instructional videos to teach pole dance exercises.

In modern day, pole dance and fitness classes are held in private studios, academies, and gym facilities worldwide, providing guidance in the practice of this discipline, as well as workshops and programs for specific and general training on the pole. Being a discipline combining Chinese circus performance, ancient Indian traditional performance, and dance and fitness skills, pole dance has grown into an internationally recognized activity for men and women alike, participating in high-standard competitions in many countries. Organizations such as the International Pole Dance and Fitness Association (IPDFA) and the International Pole Sports Federation (IPSF) are working hard to make pole dance an official part of the world's major sports competition, the Olympics.

POLE DANCE ADVANTAGES AND BENEFITS

Motivation and variety: There is a large number of moves and acrobatic tricks in pole dance and different skills to be improved for each according to their level of complexity. This guarantees the performers have a variety of challenges throughout the process, and does away with tedious, repetitive routines thereby highly increasing their motivation in each session.

Flexibility: Pole dance improves flexibility and joint mobility, as many tricks and stunts require a wide range of movements and splits. Stretching exercises prepare the body to achieve a safe and progressive improvement of performance. It is important to develop flexibility skills in a cautious manner to avoid injuries.

Self-confidence: Pole dance allows challengers to motivate themselves while observing the natural results of their performance. Seeing direct results increases expectations for new challenges with a higher level of complexity.

Suitable for all: One of the best attributes of pole dance practice is that reaches all kinds of individuals that wish to improve their lifestyle and develop new skills by practicing a sport or physical activity. Regardless of age, body structure, physical characteristics, background, or sports experience, skills will improve progressively.

Toning: Pole dance develops muscle tissue in specific areas, such as biceps, triceps, legs, glutes, hips, chest, shoulders, abdominals, and back, increasing strength while performing numerous exercises using the challenger's body weight. It also improves physical endurance and respiratory system function, and increases body stamina. With the intensity of pole dance conditioning and cardiovascular and isometric exercises, performers perceive noticeable changes regarding weight and fat reduction.

Posture: Pole dance training improves posture and body alignment by teaching performers to distribute their weight and support on muscles and ligaments in the course of each movement.

Neurological: Through the performance of sports drills and high-intensity intervals, pole dance exercises involve body movements that stimulate the prefrontal cortex of the brain which involves complex thinking, reasoning, and multi-tasking abilities, as well as problem-solving skills and attention. Various stretching exercises are similar to those found in yoga; relaxing involves the frontal lobe of the brain, which integrates thoughts and emotions. The parietal lobe is one of the most important for visual and spatial processing for all pole dance exercises. Finally, all aerobic exercises involve the hippocampus which is in charge of memory, and required for remembering the various movements, sequence of steps, and dance routines.

Stress release and expression: Dance has proven to be a most successful therapeutic tool for physical, emotional, and psychological improvement through body language, communication, and expression. Aerobic exercises stimulate the release of endorphins in the bloodstream, causing a euphoric reaction and a state of physical, mental, and emotional well-being.

Health prevention: Aerobic activities strengthen the heart and improve the respiratory system, decreasing the probability of heart disease. With the execution of different pole dance exercises, skin elasticity increases, preventing varicose vessels and osteoporosis. It has also proven to be very effective in the pre- and post-maternity process, reinforcing back and abdominal muscles.

Coordination and balance: Pole dance is intimately related to movement stability and control, through the mental and physical realization and performance of each exercise; a challenger's improvement is based on different aspects, such as body position, strength focus, weight distribution, support, and grip, as well as momentum.

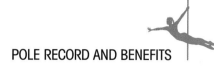

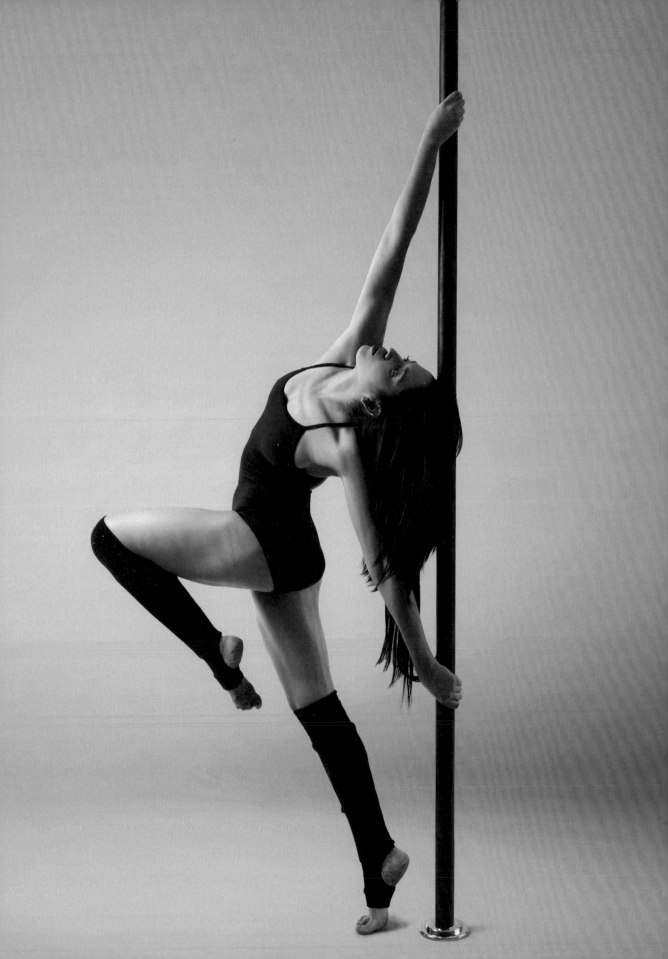

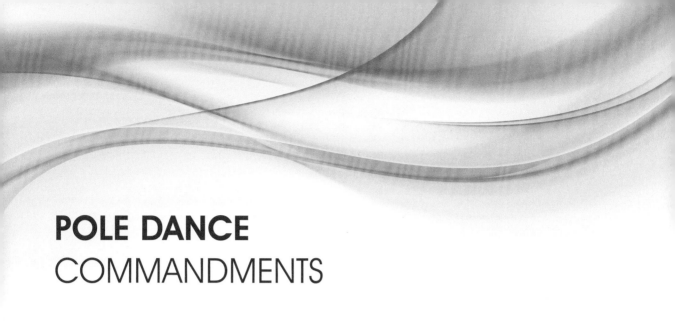

POLE DANCE
COMMANDMENTS

Warm up and stretch: The importance of proper warm-ups and stretches should not be overlooked. In order to reduce the risk of injury and fatigue, begin each pole session by performing a full-body stretch and then move on to the set of workout exercises of your preference. When the pole session concludes, select and combine your desired stretching exercises.

Check the pole's reliability: Be sure there is enough space around the pole to allow mobility, and check the pole's stability and its proper friction to the ceiling and floor.

Clean the pole: The use of isopropyl alcohol is common among performers and pole dance studios for hygiene and optimum grip purposes (sweat can be one of the main performance obstacles). However, consult with pole distributers or manufacturers for the recommended maintenance products based on the pole's material and surface qualities.

Wear proper outfits: Pole dance performance relies on stable grip and body contact to the pole. You should wear comfortable outfits that expose the proper body contact points; specifically, the arms, legs, and stomach must be uncovered in order to procure an efficiency of grip.

Have a spotter: The active participation of a certified pole dance instructor is required at all times for safety measures and proper technical instruction. In addition, training with other challengers allows information exchange, and improves social and emotional skills.

Use a crash mat: This is a valuable tool for all challengers to avoid and minimize injury risks in case of unexpected (or expected) falls from the pole. Crash mats are mainly used by beginners and by intermediate and advanced performers for tricks that involve climbing or high distance from the ground. Crash mats should not be used for grounded transitions (commonly known as floor work) or handstands to avoid any wrist injuries.

Review: Begin by practicing the last trick or spin you learned in your previous session to remind yourself of previous information and to reinforce technical and practical knowledge. This will help to improve the learning process and general optimization of the performance.

Mind technique: Each pole dance trick, spin, or movement has different characteristics, and the manner in which each of those is executed is essential. It is necessary for challengers and instructors to consider specific technical aspects, continuously gather and research new information, rehearse proper technique, acquire optimum judgment, and progressively achieve a more confident and safer performance.

Plan safety exits: While progressing on each level, the difficulty of the challenges will increase; an unexpected fall comes with no warning and often results in serious injuries. To minimize the risks, consult with the instructor for quick and safe alternative ways to exit the trick. It is recommended to begin new movements near the ground, and then move to a higher level once you are confident.

Strengthen right and left: It is common to consider one side's extremities to be stronger than the other, creating a sensation of safety and comfort while performing. This preference can be counterproductive, increasing risk of injuries and developing muscular mass unevenly. Although you may be stronger side on one side or the other, the goal is to equally and progressively prepare and train the body for the different challenges.

Stay hydrated: The quality and quantity of pole dance exercises require considerable endurance, strength, resistance, and stamina. It is important to stay hydrated before, during, and after training, and to include proper meal plans before and after your training sessions to provide the body with the energy it requires to achieve an effective performance.

Play music: It is highly recommended to play music during the execution of the exercises in order to improve cerebral stimulation, motor control functions, and emotional motivation, significantly contributing to the performer's progress.

Keep up the good work: Keeping a positive attitude will greatly contribute to the challenger's performance. It is essential to practice continuously and rigorously, maintaining focus, persistence, and motivation for the upcoming challenges and achievements. Results are a certainty.

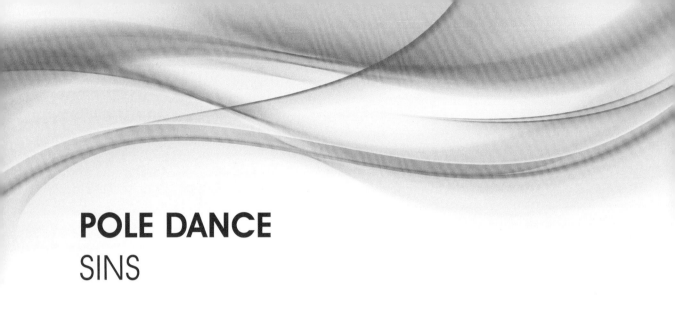

POLE DANCE
SINS

Moisturizing: This is one of the most important rules in pole dance. Do not apply body creams, oils, moistening products, or lotions that will eradicate the grip on the pole for at least 24 hours prior to the session.

Jewelry: Safety guidelines include the removal of all earrings, bracelets, rings, necklaces, piercings, or any other objects that might come into contact with the pole in order to avoid any sort of skin lacerations or damages to the pole or the jewelry itself.

Grip aids: Attempting to obtain a better grip on the pole by the regular and excessive use of different tools or products is a counterproductive and unconstructive habit which most likely minimizes skills development on the pole. It is important to progressively condition the body to obtain the appropriate strength in order to perform future high-complexity challenges, especially during the introductory phase and at the basic level.

Static or spinning poles: Both modes provide different advantages. It is recommended to practice alternating on both pole modes. Avoid becoming accustomed to a single type which restricts the skills development and progress in general.

Performing under the influence: Pole dance is a high-level physical and mental practice based on the accurate execution of acrobatic movements and aerial stunts. The use of substances such as hallucinogens, opiates, or alcohol may have debilitating effects in addition to altering senses and negatively influencing motor activity, coordination, reflexes, and judgement, resulting in serious injuries or other grave repercussions.

Haste: Rushing through the learning progression in order to get to more advanced challenges is common, especially if the desired results are not yet perceived. However, the necessary skills will improve gradually, along with patience and persistence which are fundamental and positive qualities to develop in the learning process. Basic foundations and each level's tricks pursue specific objectives, regardless of their complexity; each one is crucial for future challenges and achievements.

Injuries and overuse: Continuous training and repetitive overuse of muscles are common while performing pole dance and may lead to chronic injuries if left untreated. The most usual muscle injuries are rotator cuff and deltoid strain, wrist sprain, carpal tunnel syndrome, and hamstring, intercostal, and forearm strains. It is necessary to gradually strengthen muscles and improve flexibility by performing specific exercises and receiving proper therapeutic treatment. In case of discomfort, falls, or injuries, consult a certified physician.

Sleep and rest deprivation: Rest is fundamental for optimum brain and body functions. Sleep deprivation increases fatigue, and lowers energy and focus. During sleep and rest, the body generates a growth hormone, which contributes to tissue growth and repair, increasing vitality and positively influencing multiple aspects of the athlete's practice and performance.

Bad posture: It is crucial to maintain proper postures for each movement, trick, spin, and routine that is being performed. Each of the pole dance challenges require postures that must be constantly considered to accomplish a cautious and graceful performance, procuring long-term physical improvements.

Panic: Because pole dance is a high-risk sport involving aerial stunts and acrobatic movements, it is natural to feel pain or experience fear and panic, leading to a sudden pole release and risking the challenger's own safety as well as that of the spotter. In case of difficulties, it is recommended to practice different breathing techniques and to use crash mats and safety exit procedures.

Frustration: Emotional dissatisfaction increases stress and demotivation, leading to general disappointment. This negatively influences the learning process and, eventually, the performance. Each challenger works at a different pace, and has their own individual characteristics, strengths, and weaknesses; it is important to persevere and remember that all achievements require persistence and determination. Optimum results will be revealed in time and success will overcome.

Neglecting the weak side: Performing pole dance stunts and spins on a preferable side of the body is a counterproductive practice; it weakens the extremities and limits the challenger's expertise and conditioning process.

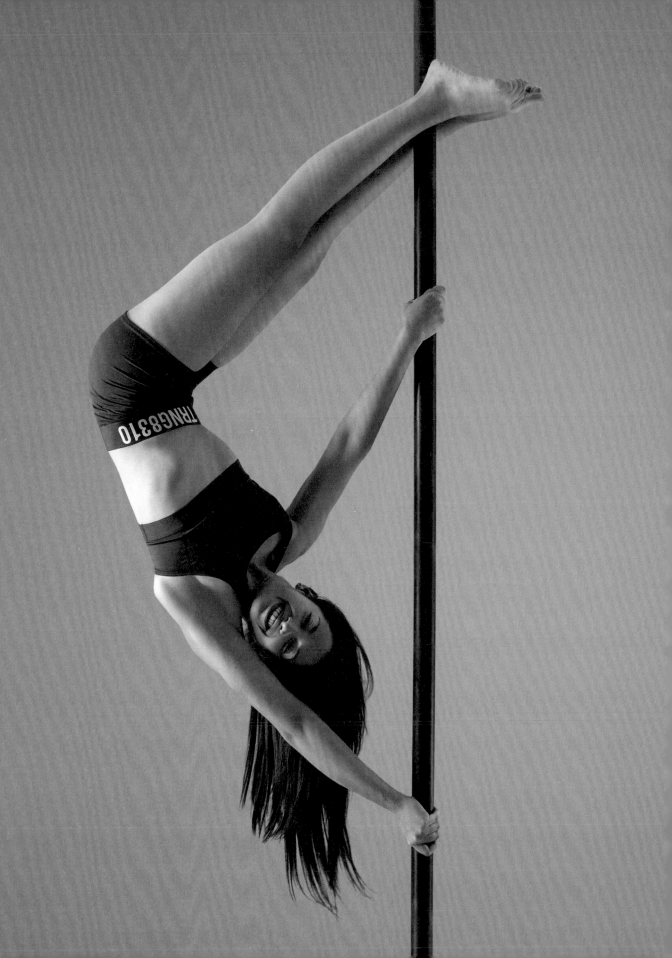

HOW TO USE
THIS GUIDE

The pole dance and fitness guide is structured as a rigorous program for each of your sessions using the following steps:

1. Review the sections on pole commandments and sins.

2. Complete a selection of the pre-workout stretches.

3. Select and perform one of the workout sets.

4. Complement the workout set with:

   a. Pole warms-ups

   b. Conditioning postural exercises

   c. Transitional movements

   d. Climbs

   e. Shoulder mounts

   f. Handstands

   g. Latest trick or routine

8. Search the pole program for the trick you worked on during your last session and, if achieved, move on to the next challenge.

9. Select stretching exercises to begin relaxation.

Let's get started!

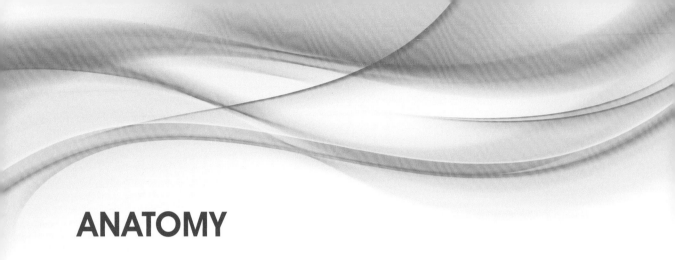

ANATOMY

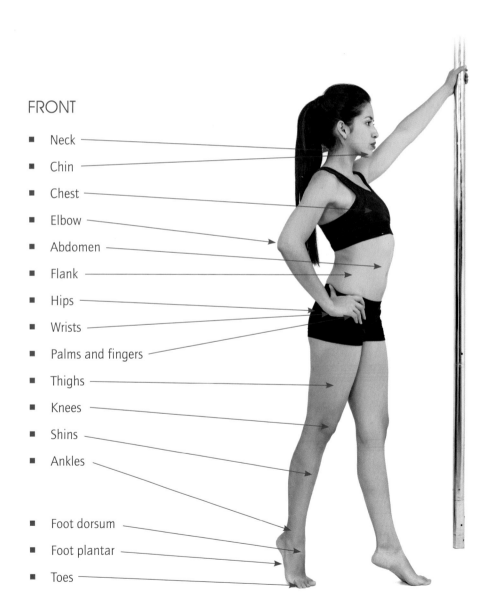

FRONT

- Neck
- Chin
- Chest
- Elbow
- Abdomen
- Flank
- Hips
- Wrists
- Palms and fingers
- Thighs
- Knees
- Shins
- Ankles

- Foot dorsum
- Foot plantar
- Toes

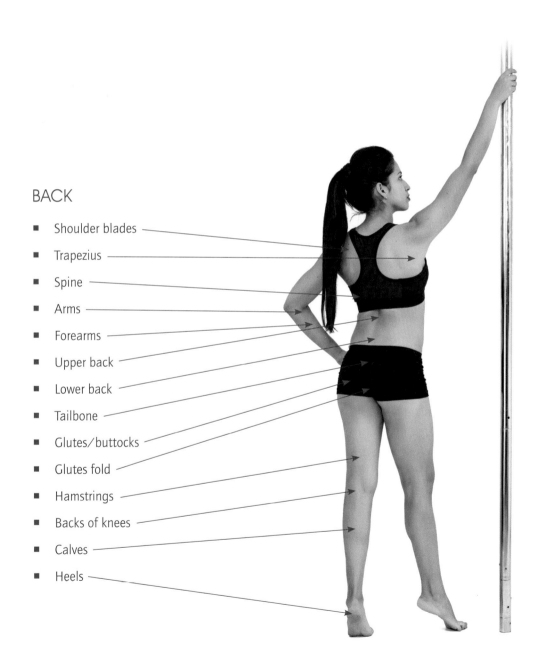

BACK

- Shoulder blades
- Trapezius
- Spine
- Arms
- Forearms
- Upper back
- Lower back
- Tailbone
- Glutes/buttocks
- Glutes fold
- Hamstrings
- Backs of knees
- Calves
- Heels

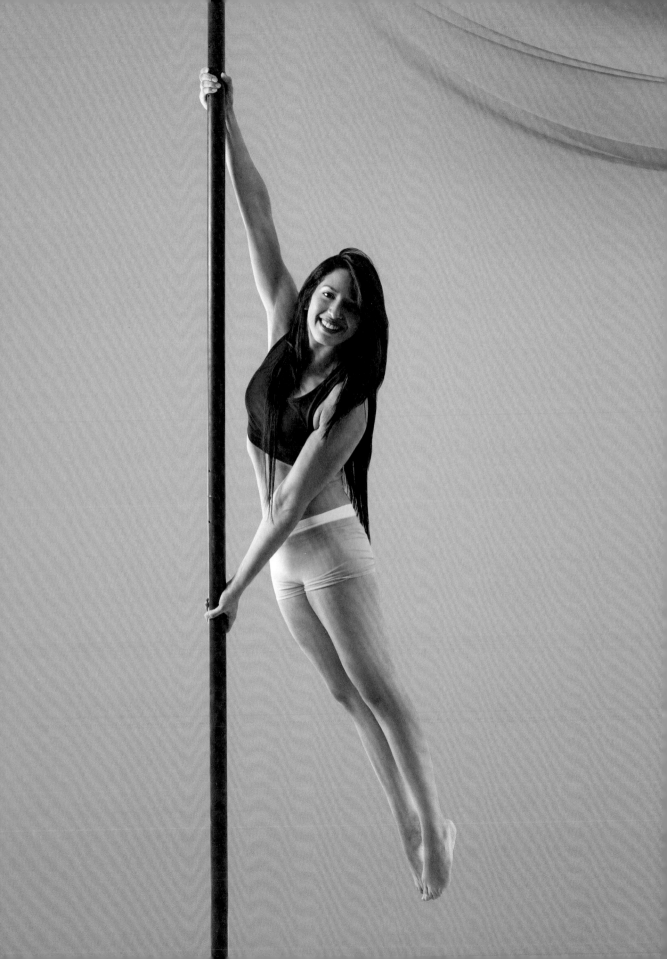

CHAPTER 1
POSITIONS AND POLE PRINCIPLES

CHAPTER 1
POSITIONS AND POLE PRINCIPLES

The positions of the body, arms, and legs, along with the technical understanding of each of the movements executed, are essential for an appropriate and safe performance in pole dance. Each pole dance stunt has different characteristics, and the manner in which each of those is executed is essential. It is vital to consider and progressively obtain the understanding of the practical and technical aspects of pole dance: the best way to perform each trick; the correct body alignment to ensure the optimal placement of different body parts; and the optimal foot placement to obtain a visually appealing performance, to improve grip, or to secure the body position on the pole.

Pole dance and fitness is based on various physics principles, such as equilibrium, momentum, friction, gravity, rotational inertia, and angular velocity. Angular momentum refers to the performer's movements and the forces applied while spinning around the pole, depending on the stunt or exercise to be performed. To gain momentum, dancers extend and swing the extremities around the pole before performing the spin or trick. It is important to remember that while tricks are executed on the spinning pole and while challengers apply a certain amount of strength to gain momentum, the pole will always spin faster while the challenger's extremities are closer to it; conversely, the further from the pole the challenger is, the slower the spinning velocity will be. All pole dance climbs are subject to gravity and friction principles involving significant motor control; sliding down the pole from high levels and performing multiple stunts also depends on relevant factors on the frictional force such as the pole's characteristics and the challenger's grip. The centrifugal force causes the sensation of being drawn away from the pole while the centripetal force attracts the body toward it. Body balance is also an important aspect in pole dance; most movements require rotation and inversion of the body in addition to speed and the performer's individual characteristics. Each stunt and movement demands different strength points and an intensity focused on the stability of each body part and weight distribution. One of the basic pole principles emphasizes the pull and push actions, in which each extremity or body part performs either of the tasks. It is common to apply this force on hand grips, where the upper hand performs a pulling action on the pole and the lower one pushes the body away from it.

General and specific performance skills will be developed continuously and progressively for the duration of the learning process. Gathering and continuously researching information from challengers and instructors is necessary for an enriched experience and a better performance.

BODY POSITIONS

- Inverted
- Standing
- Horizontal

HAND GRIPS AND ARM POSITIONS

- One-hand basic grip
- Two-handed split grip
- Two-handed full-bracket split grip
- One-hand down grip
- Two-handed half grip
- Baseball grip
- One-hand strong hold
- Two-handed strong hold
- Forearm grip
- Two-handed partial split grip
- One-hand back support
- Two-handed baseball back support
- One-hand down baseball grip
- Two-handed twisted grip
- Two-handed flag grip
- One-hand twisted grip
- Two-handed reverse grab
- Two-handed half-inverted grip
- Two-handed iguana grip

- One-hand bridge arch
- One-hand cup grip
- Two-handed double bridge arch
- Two-handed cup grip
- Two-handed basic cup
- Two-handed basic princess grip
- Two-handed true grip
- Two-handed princess grip
- Two-handed flip grip
- One-hand claw grip
- One-hand elbow grip
- Two-handed double elbow and variation
- Underarm grip
- Two-handed elbow split grip
- Two-handed archer elbow grip
- Armpit grip
- Two-handed embrace hang
- Two-handed crossed grip

LEG POSITIONS

- Straddle
- Crossed
- Scissors
- Stag/double attitude
- Split

- Tuck
- Fang
- Pike
- Passé
- Pencil

BODY POSITIONS

Body positions are based on three basic poses: inversions, stands, and the horizontal line of the body. If the back and shoulders are positioned above the waist, it is a standing position; if the waist is above the back and shoulders, it is an inverted position; and if the legs, waist, and back are aligned and parallel to the floor, it is a horizontal position. Exercises are characterized by which extremities are closest to the pole. The importance of technical aspects must not be overlooked: body position, grip, muscle contractions, extension or flexion, and pressure points, as well as safety measures and individual capabilities. Pole dance is as much an athletic activity as it is an artistic one. There must be a balance between the precision and accuracy required when performing the different movements and routines and the creative expression of the performer for motivational purposes, effective progress, and expected accomplishments.

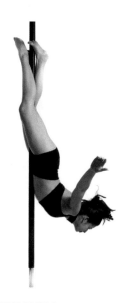

INVERSION

Basic inversion into aerial leg hold to inverted crucifix.

Grip: Ankle, knees, and thighs

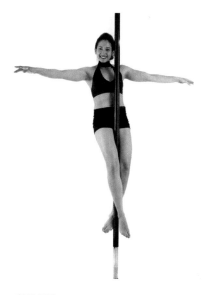

STAND

Basic climb technique to aerial leg hold.

Grip: Ankles, knees, thighs,
and core muscles

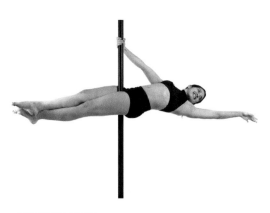

HORIZONTAL

Basic pole sit to plank supported by the upper hand.

Grip: Thighs, single hand, shoulders, and core muscles

HAND GRIPS AND ARM POSITIONS

Every pole dance trick is followed by a series of arm positions, movements, and grips; this is followed by transitions from one trick to the next that require a variety of additional postures and subsequent grips. There are also many pole tricks and movements that don't use hand grips and instead depend on support from other body parts. It is crucial to identify the requirements of each trick and recognize the correct body friction points for a more accurate and safer performance. The pull and push actions—in which the upper hand applies a pulling force from the pole and the lower hand applies a pushing force to it—are some of the most important principles of pole dance, bearing in mind the distribution of weight and support on the arms, body balance, and duration and speed of each transitional movement and trick. During the learning process, experience will guarantee increasing confidence, and self-realized techniques distinctive to each challenger according to individual characteristics will allow for the achievement of different purposes and eventually an improved performance.

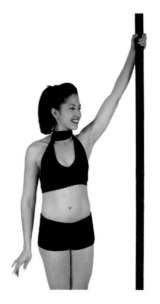

ONE-HAND BASIC GRIP

One arm extends higher overhead with a full grip (i.e., thumb facing fingers).

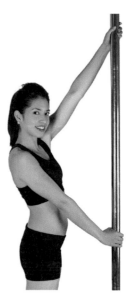

TWO-HANDED SPLIT GRIP

One arm extends higher overhead with the opposite arm at hip level with a full grip (i.e., thumb facing fingers).

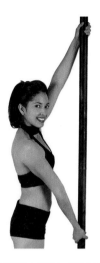

TWO-HANDED FULL-BRACKET SPLIT GRIP

One arm extends overhead with the palm facing sideways while the other arm extends down to pubic bone level with the palm facing away.

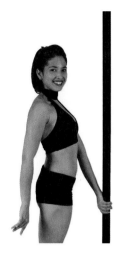

ONE-HAND DOWN GRIP

One arm extends down to mid-thigh level with a full grip and the palm facing away from the body.

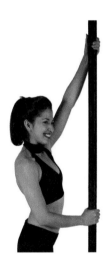

TWO-HANDED HALF GRIP

One arm extends overhead while the other arm is stuck into the body with the elbow flexed to 90 degrees and the forearm just under the rib cage. Both hands use a full grip.

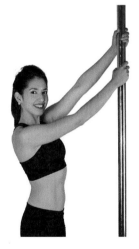

BASEBALL GRIP

With the body facing the pole, both arms extend to head level and the hands use a full grip (i.e., thumbs facing fingers).

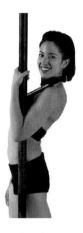

ONE-HAND STRONG HOLD

With the body positioned sideways to pole, the pole is anchored under the arm with the biceps stuck into it, the elbow flexed, and the hand using a full grip at ear level.

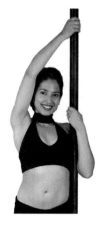

TWO-HANDED STRONG HOLD

With the body positioned sideways to pole, the near arm assumes a strong hold grip. The far arm is extended or bent overhead with the forearm facing the forehead and the palm facing backward.

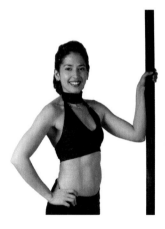

FOREARM GRIP

With the body positioned sideways to the pole, one arm extends to front at shoulder level with the elbow flexed to 90 degrees. The forearm is supported on the pole, with the hand using a full grip.

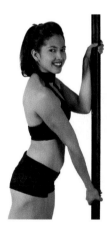

TWO-HANDED PARTIAL SPLIT GRIP

With the body facing the pole, one arm flexes to 90 degrees with the elbow at shoulder level, the forearm supported on the pole, and the hand holding with a full grip at head level. The other arm extends down to pubic bone level with the palm facing away from the body.

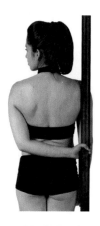

ONE-HAND BACK SUPPORT

With the body positioned sideways to the pole, the far arm wraps behind the back and grabs the pole just above the hip with a full grip and the palm facing backwards. The near arm remains free.

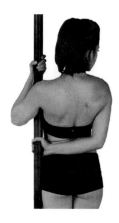

TWO-HANDED BASEBALL BACK SUPPORT

With the body positioned sideways to the pole and the near arm using a baseball grip, the far arm wraps behind the back and the hand grasps the pole just above the hip with a full grip, palm facing backwards.

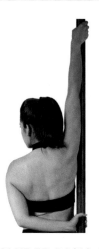

TWO-HANDED BASIC SUPPORT

With the body positioned sideways to the pole, the near arm extends overhead and the hand grasps the pole with a full grip, palm facing forward. The far arm wraps horizontally around the back and the hand grasps the pole just above the hip with a full grip, palm facing backwards.

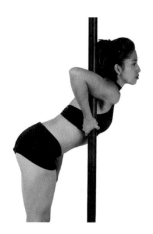

ONE-HAND DOWN BASEBALL GRIP

With the body positioned sideways to the pole and the pole anchored under the near arm, the shoulder is extended back, the elbow is flexed and pointing back at shoulder level, and the hand grips the pole at the lower rib level, palm facing forward.

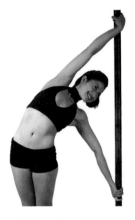

TWO-HANDED TWISTED GRIP

With the body positioned sideways to the pole, the near arm extends downward to mid-thigh level and the hand grasps the pole with a full grip, palm facing backwards. The far arm extends to the pole, twists around it, and uses a full grip with the palm facing backwards.

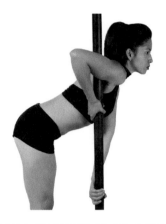

TWO-HANDED FLAG GRIP

With the body positioned sideways to the pole and the near arm positioned in the one-hand down baseball grip position, the far arm extends down and grips the pole at knee level, palm facing forward.

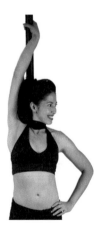

ONE-HAND TWISTED GRIP

With the body facing away from the pole, the far arm extends behind the head and the hand twists around the pole to grasp it with a full grip.

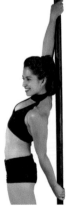

TWO-HANDED REVERSE GRAB

With the body facing away from pole, one arm extends down and behind, just below glutes with the palm facing backwards. The other arm extends overhead and twists behind the body with the palm facing to the side and both hands using a full grip.

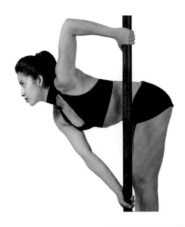

TWO-HANDED HALF-INVERTED GRIP

With the upper body positioned sideways to the pole, the far arm extends down with the palm facing the body at knee level. The near arm extends up behind the body with the elbow flexed to 90 degrees and the hand facing body (both with a full grip).

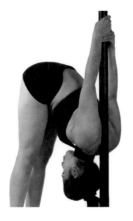

TWO-HANDED IGUANA GRIP

With the body facing the pole, the head inverted, and the upper back supported on the pole, both arms extend up slightly higher than hip level, and the hands grasp the pole with a full grip.

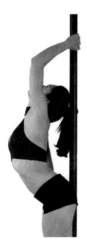

ONE-HAND BRIDGE ARCH

With the body arched out and facing away from pole, one arm extends up behind the body with the elbow flexed at head level and the hand grasping the pole slightly above the head with a full grip.

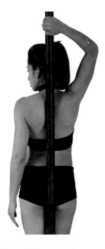

ONE-HAND CUP GRIP

With the body facing away and supported by the pole, one arm extends up with the elbow flexed to 90 degrees and the hand grasps the pole with an opened fist grip.

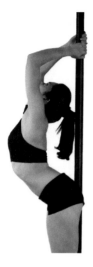

TWO-HANDED DOUBLE BRIDGE ARCH

With the body arched out and facing away from the pole, both arms extend up behind the body with the elbows flexed at head level and the hands slightly passing each other above the head with the palms opposite each other.

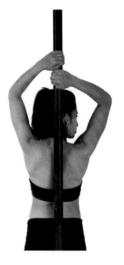

TWO-HANDED CUP GRIP

With the back of the body stuck into the pole, both arms extend up with the elbows flexed to 90 degrees and the hands grasp the pole with an opened fist grip.

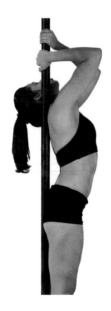

TWO-HANDED BASIC CUP

With the body facing away from the pole and one shoulder supported, the neck extends back with the head past the pole. One arm extends up with the elbow flexed and the hand in a cup grip at ear level, palm facing forward. The other arm extends up with the elbow flexed and the full grip is reversed, with the hand just past the other one and the palm facing sideways.

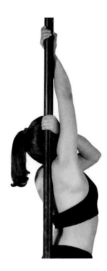

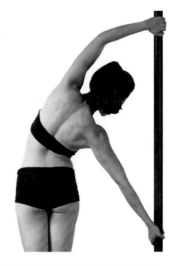

TWO-HANDED BASIC PRINCESS GRIP

With the body facing away from pole and the head past the pole, one arm extends up high with a twisted full grip while the other one wraps around the neck, holding the pole at ear level with a full grip.

TWO-HANDED TRUE GRIP

With the body positioned sideways to the pole, the far arm reaches up overhead with the elbow slightly flexed and the hand in a cup grip facing forward. The near arm extends down to mid-thigh level with the hand in a full grip and the palm facing sideways.

TWO-HANDED PRINCESS GRIP

With the body facing away from the pole, one arm extends up with the elbow flexed to 90 degrees and the hand in a cup grip behind the head. The other arm extends up high and the hand uses a twisted grip to grasp the pole.

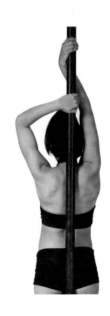

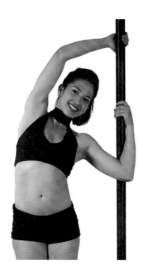

TWO-HANDED FLIP GRIP

With the body positioned sideways to the pole and the near shoulder extended before the pole, flex the elbow and hook into the pole with the hand back in a full grip. The far arm extends up with the elbow flexed, the forearm just above the head, the hand in a cup grip, and the palm facing forward.

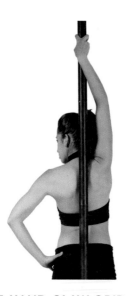

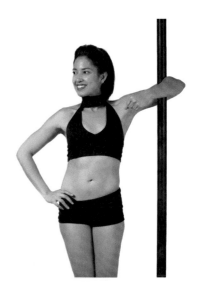

ONE-HAND CLAW GRIP

With the body facing away from pole, one arm extends up high and twists around the pole. The hand grasps the pole between the index and middle fingers with the palm facing forward.

ONE-HAND ELBOW GRIP

With the body positioned sideways to the pole, the near arm extends to the side and behind it. The elbow should be flexed higher than shoulder level and hooked around the pole.

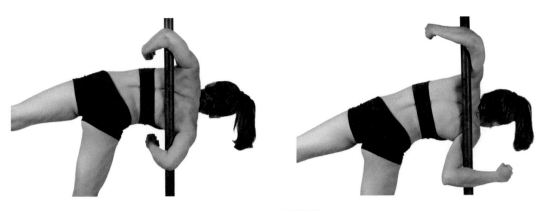

TWO-HANDED DOUBLE ELBOW AND VARIATION

With the body facing away from the pole, both arms extend behind and the elbows flex, pointing back and hooking around the pole. Hands should be free and facing forward.

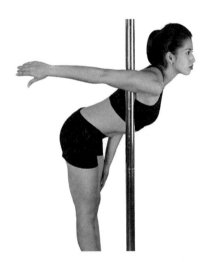

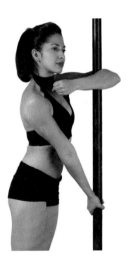

UNDERARM GRIP

With the body positioned sideways to the pole, the pole is anchored under the near arm which is fully extended at elbow or shoulder level and pointing backwards.

TWO-HANDED ELBOW SPLIT GRIP

With the body facing sideways to the pole, the near arm extends to the side and the elbow flexes above shoulder level, hooking around the pole. The far arm extends down with the palm facing away at pubic bone level. The hand should grasp the pole with a full grip.

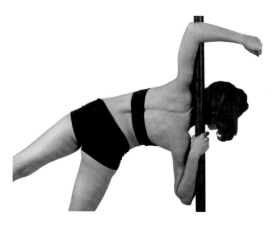

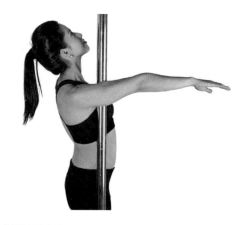

TWO-HANDED ARCHER ELBOW GRIP

One arm extends behind and over the pole with the elbow flexed and hooked into it. The other arm wraps behind under the pole with the elbow flexed and the hand grasps the pole with a full grip at neck level.

ARMPIT GR

With the body facing sideways to the pole, anchor the pole under the arm and fully extend it forward.

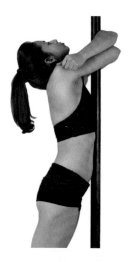

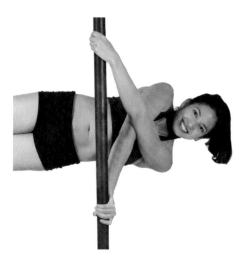

TWO-HANDED EMBRACE HANG

With the body facing the pole and both arms extended to the front, the elbows flex with one just past the other higher than shoulder level and hook around the pole. Palms are either free or hugging the shoulders.

TWO-HANDED CROSSED GRIP

With the body facing the pole and the arms extended and crossed over, the hands grasp the pole with a full grip and the palms facing the body.

LEG POSITIONS

Pole dance performance is made up of diverse body movements in which each body part has a specific task. The legs are an important part of these movements and there are a number of positions to be considered. Most tricks have basic characteristics and mandatory requirements for best execution, bearing in mind technical aspects of the trick and each position's visual appeal (e.g., complete leg extension or flexion, grips, and friction on the pole). In order to achieve an optimum performance, leg muscles must be contracted at all times, maintaining flexed plantars and pointed toes throughout the execution of movements and positions, specifically following the different exercise indications and suggested guidelines.

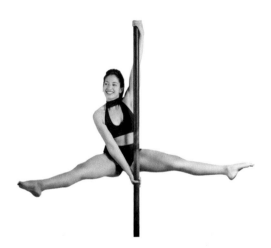

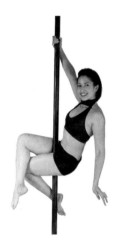

STRADDLE

With the body facing the pole, both thighs are flexed wider than the hips and are abducted with the pole centralized. Knees are fully extended.

CROSSED

With the body facing sideways to the pole, both thighs flex to 90 degrees at the hip and cross over. Knees are flexed.

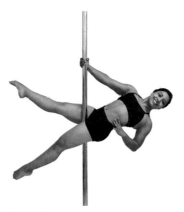

SCISSORS

With the body facing the pole and the pole positioned between the thighs, both thighs are flexed to 90 degrees at the hip and are adducted. Knees fully extend forward and both thighs press against the pole. The upper leg is elevated and the lower leg is depressed in the opposite direction.

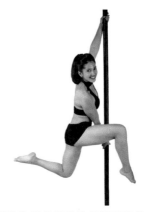

STAG/DOUBLE ATTITUDE

With the body facing the pole, one thigh is flexed to 90 degrees at the hip and the opposite knee is flexed back at the thigh. Both knees are flexed to 90 degrees and the pole is centralized.

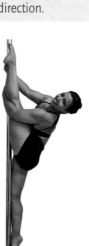

SPLIT

With the body facing the pole, one thigh flexed at the hip, the knee extended, and toes pointed, the other thigh extends down along with the knee. Both thighs are supported on the pole.

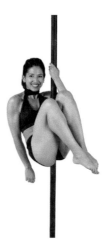

TUCK

With the body positioned sideways to the pole, both thighs are flexed at the hip and the knees are flexed at chest level.

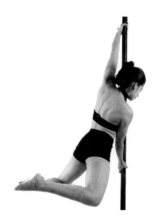

FANG

Both thighs extend back, laterally rotated slightly wider than the hip. Both knees are flexed to 90 degrees and the toes are in contact with each other.

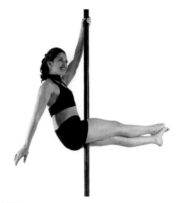

PIKE

With the pole between the thighs as the body faces it, both thighs flex to 90 degrees at the hip and are adducted. Knees fully extend forward and the ankles are crossed.

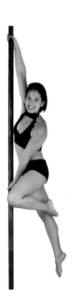

PASSÉ

With the body facing the pole, one thigh extends down parallel to it with the front of the thigh facing forward. The other thigh flexes to 90 degrees at the hip and is laterally rotated with a flexed knee.

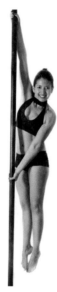

PENCIL

With the body facing the pole, both thighs extend down parallel to it and face sideways.

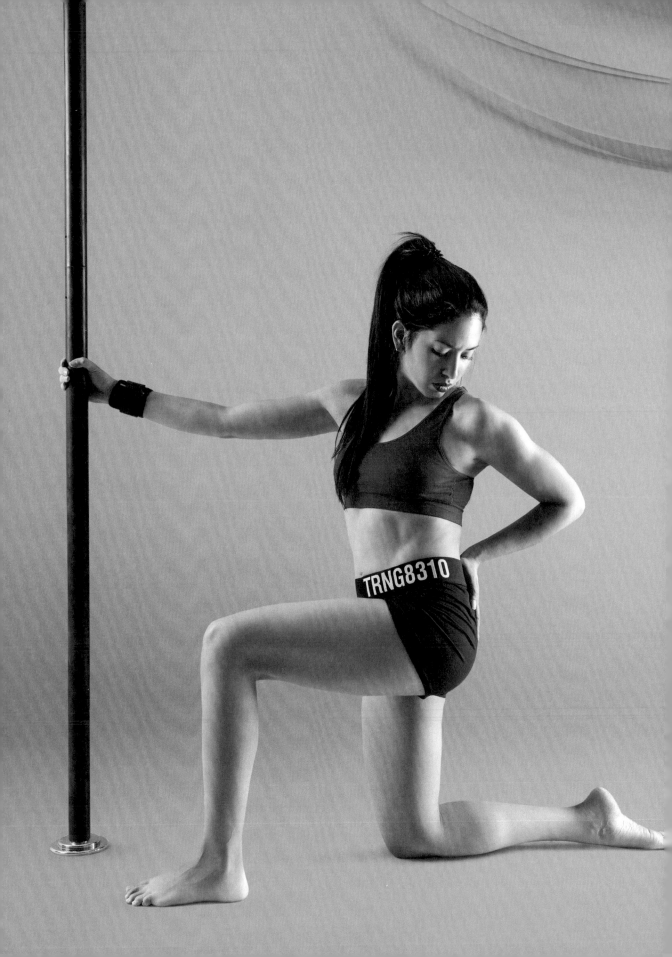

CHAPTER 2
PRE-WORKOUT STRETCHING

CHAPTER 2
PRE-WORKOUT STRETCHING

In order to provide readers with a comprehensive guide to the activities performed before each pole session, a variety of stretching exercises to complement the workout sets have been selected to be combined freely by challengers as needed.

Stretching improves flexibility skills through the execution of numerous exercises and gentle stationary movements, activating major body joints in preparation for higher intensity training. These stretches may target multiple or specific areas, improving joint mobility through a full range of motion, easing muscle tension, decreasing fatigue, and resulting in circulation, muscle coordination, and overall physical performance improvements.

Selected stretches should relate to the stunts that will be practiced; it is also recommended to cover upper- and lower-body stretches to minimize injury risks, maintaining positions for a minimum of 10-15 seconds and doing four to five repetitions on each side of the body. You should gently stretch the muscle further with each repetition, but there is no need for drastic movements or intense pressure. It is common to feel sensitivity while performing certain movements, but challengers and trainers must be careful to distinguish between the common slight discomfort given by pressure applied to the exercised area and noticeable pain, which is certainly counterproductive. It is also a good idea to wear an appropriate warm-up outfit to cover exposed areas (e.g., leg warmers, tights, sweat pants, or thin sweaters).

Proper breathing technique is vital to the pursuit of an effective stretch, optimizing blood circulation and significantly improving the exercise's results. Holding your breath while executing these exercises is common, but it must be avoided in order to achieve positive effects and outcomes.

Bear in mind that the purpose of this basic stretching routine is the execution of moderate physical effort while avoiding extreme exhaustion, considering the intensive conditioning exercises (i.e., workout sets) are also to be performed in the same session.

Skill development will improve through continuous repetition and training a minimum of three to four times per week, depending on the challenger's individual qualities, capabilities, and performance. A minimum of ten to fifteen repetitions on each side of the body is recommended.

It is highly recommended that challengers consult a certified physician before attempting to perform this activity, during training, and in the case of discomfort of any sort.

UPPER-BODY MOBILITY AND STRETCH EXERCISES

- Neck flexion and extension
- Overhead arm pull
- Head semi-circle
- Neck rotation stretch
- Neck side stretch
- Shoulder stretch
- Up and down shoulder shrugs
- Shoulder rotations
- Shoulder stretch
- Abdominal stretch
- Side stretch

- Chest rotations
- Waist side to side
- Hip rotations
- Waist rotations
- Waist and lower-limb rotations
- Back rotation stretch
- Forward bend stretch
- Bending windmill stretch
- Double-arm inverted stretch
- Wrist rotation

LOWER-BODY MOBILITY AND STRETCH EXERCISES

- Standing hamstring stretch
- Calf stretch
- Quadriceps stretch
- Wide-leg forward bend
- Wide-leg forward bend (ankle pull)
- Wide leg sideways bend
- Lateral hip flexors and extensors
- Internal and external knee rotations
- Kneeling hip flexor
- Seated hamstring stretch
- Butterfly stretch
- Supine piriformis stretch
- Supine leg stretch

- Supine hamstring stretch
- Grounded back bend
- Grounded hip stretch
- Extended lunge stretch
- Cat and cow stretch
- Hip flexors stretch
- Bow pose
- Forward lean straddle stretch
- Sideways lean straddle stretch
- Hyperextension
- Lying abdominal stretch
- Modified downward dog
- Downward dog position

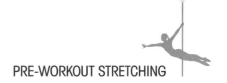

UPPER-BODY MOBILITY AND STRETCH EXERCISES

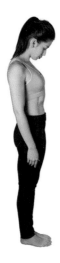
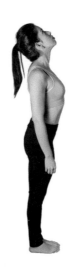

NECK FLEXION AND EXTENSION

Stand with the hands extended comfortably along the sides. Gently tilt the head forward and then backward to stretch. Repeat 2 to 3 times.

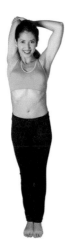
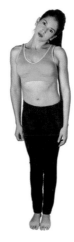

OVERHEAD ARM PULL

Raise the right arm over the head with the elbow pointing up. Pull the elbow down toward the opposite side with the opposite hand. Repeat 2 to 3 times on each side.

HEAD SEMI-CIRCLE

With the head and back in an upright position, rotate the neck to the right and left sides. Use a semi-circle movement to return to the starting position. Repeat 5 to 10 times.

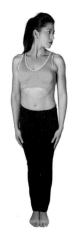

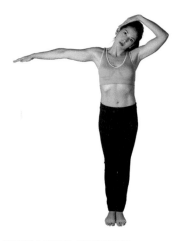

NECK ROTATION STRETCH

Standing in an upright position, rotate the neck to the left and right sides. Gently extend the neck backward and flex forward. Finally, rotate the head from left to right. Repeat in the opposite direction. Repeat 5 to 10 times.

NECK SIDE STRETCH

Standing in an upright position, bend the head to one side. To increase the stretch, place the opposite hand over the head and gently pull it further to the side. Repeat on the opposite side. Repeat 5 to 10 times.

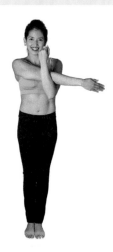

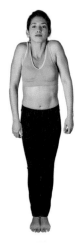

SHOULDER STRETCH

Standing in an upright position, the arm fully extends across the body and the opposite hand holds the upper arm to flex the shoulder. Hold the position for 30 seconds before repeating on the opposite side.

UP AND DOWN SHOULDER SHRUGS

Standing in an upright position, shrug the shoulders up and down. Repeat 10 to 15 times.

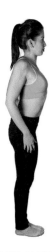 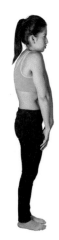

SHOULDER ROTATIONS

Rotate the shoulders backward, then reverse the movement, rotating shoulders forward. Repeat 10 to 15 times in each direction.

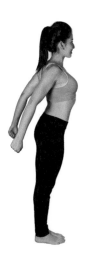 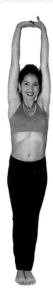

SHOULDER STRETCH (ANTERIOR CAPSULE)

Stand in an upright position with the arms along the sides. Extend backward through the full range of motion. Hold the position for 15 to 20 seconds.

ABDOMINAL STRETCH

Raise the arms over head, interlock the fingers, and slightly stretch upward. Hold the position for 10 seconds.

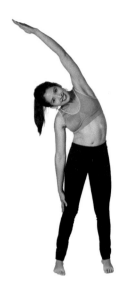

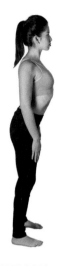

SIDE STRETCH

Stand with feet hip-distance apart, maintaining centralized hips. Bend the torso sideways, sliding the hand down to knee level. The opposite arm fully extends overhead. Repeat the exercise on the opposite side.

CHEST ROTATIONS

Keep the waist in a fixed position. Move the chest forward, squeezing the shoulder blades together. Tilting the trunk to one side, move the chest backward, rounding the shoulders forward and then tilting the trunk to the opposite side. Continuously rotate the trunk.

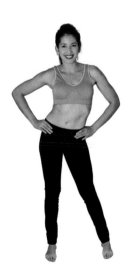

WAIST SIDE TO SIDE

With the hands at waist level, push the pelvis sideways. Repeat 10 to 15 times in both directions.

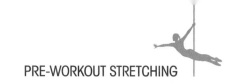

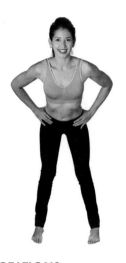
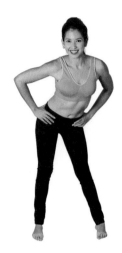

HIP ROTATIONS

Stand with the legs slightly wider than hip-distance apart and rotate the hips.
Repeat 10 to 15 times in both directions.

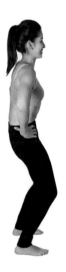
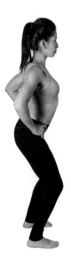

WAIST ROTATIONS

Stand with feet hip-distance apart. Flex the hips and knees to rotate the waist anteriorly, laterally, and posteriorly, then reverse. Continuously rotate the waist 10 to 15 times in each direction.

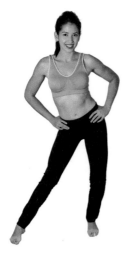

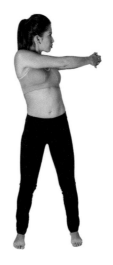

WAIST AND LOWER-LIMB ROTATIONS

Tilt the trunk sideways, slightly flex the knees, and rotate the hips anteriorly, laterally, and posteriorly. Repeat on the opposite side.

BACK ROTATION STRETCH

Standing in an upright position with the arms extended forward and fingers interlocked together, rotate the arms and head to one side, keeping the elbows slightly bent. Maintain centered hips.
Repeat 5 to 10 times on both sides.

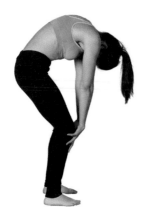

FORWARD BEND STRETCH

Standing in an upright position, slightly bend the knees and lean the trunk forward, bringing the chin to the sternal notch to stretch the back muscles. Return to the starting position and repeat 10 times.

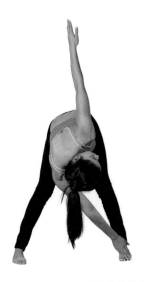

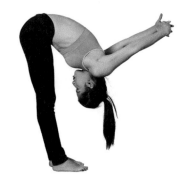

BENDING WINDMILL STRETCH

Stand in an upright position. Lean forward and extend one arm toward the opposite foot. Raise the other arm while maintaining eye contact with it. Repeat the exercise 10 times on each side.

DOUBLE-ARM INVERTED STRETCH

Stand in an upright position. Extend the arms backward and interlock the fingers. Slightly lean forward, raising the arms away from the trunk.

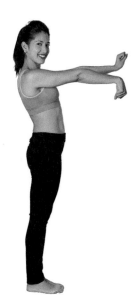

WRIST ROTATION

Standing in an upright position with the arms fully extended forward, perform slight wrist rotations in both directions.

LOWER-BODY MOBILITY AND STRETCH EXERCISES

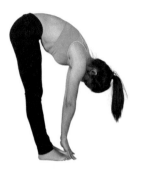

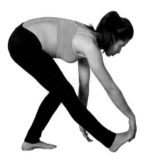

STANDING HAMSTRING STRETCH

Stand in an upright position. Lean forward and reach for the feet. Maintain knee extension and hold position.

CALF STRETCH

Stand in an upright position and flex the left knee. The opposite leg takes a step forward, maintaining knee extension and foot dorsiflexion with heel-to-ground contact. Lean forward and reach toward the dorsiflexed foot. Hold this position for 10 seconds. Repeat the exercise with the opposite leg.

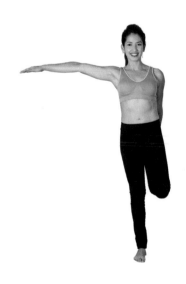

QUADRICEPS STRETCH

Stand in an upright position. Flex one knee backward and hold the ankle. Abduct opposite arm to maintain balance.

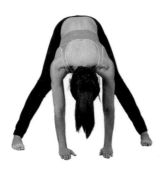

WIDE-LEG FORWARD BEND

Stand in an upright position with feet wider than hip-distance apart. Maintaining centralized hips, lean forward and rest the palms on the ground. Back and arms should be extended.

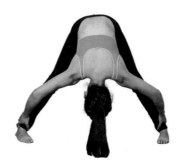

WIDE-LEG FORWARD BEND (ANKLE PULL)

Stand in an upright position with feet wider than hip-distance apart. Maintaining centralized hips, lean forward to grasp the ankles and slightly pull. Elbows remain flexed.

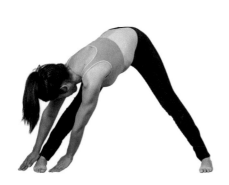

WIDE-LEG SIDEWAYS BEND

Stand in an upright position with feet wider than hip-distance apart. Maintaining centralized hips and extending the back, lean the trunk toward one leg. Reach both hands out toward the foot and gently bounce. Repeat on the opposite side.

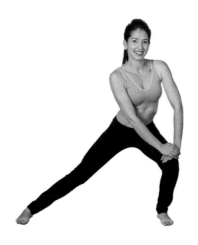

LATERAL HIP FLEXORS AND EXTENSORS

Stand in an upright position with feet wider than hip-distance apart. Keeping the hips centralized, flex one knee and lean the torso toward the leg. Maintain back alignment and support both hands on the knee. Repeat with the opposite leg.

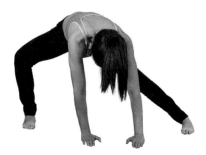 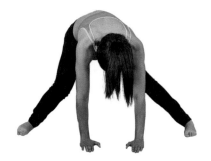

INTERNAL AND EXTERNAL KNEE ROTATIONS

Standing in an upright position with feet wider than hip-distance apart, lean forward to rest palms on the ground. Maintain elbow extension and back alignment. With hands and hips centralized, rotate the knee out and in. Repeat with the opposite leg.

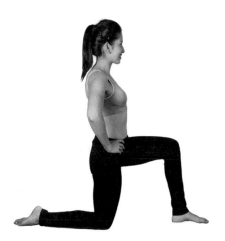

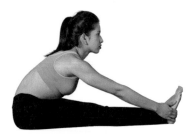

KNEELING HIP FLEXOR

Stand in an upright position. Flex the hip and knee to step forward and kneel on the opposite leg. Press the hips forward while maintaining an upright posture.

SEATED HAMSTRING STRETCH

Sit comfortably and maintain upright posture with the legs extended. Bend the torso over the thighs and hold this position for 15-20 seconds

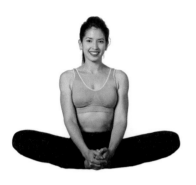

BUTTERFLY STRETCH

Sit upright, maintaining contact between the soles of the feet and with the thighs abducted. Lean forward and hold this position while gently pressing the knees to the ground.

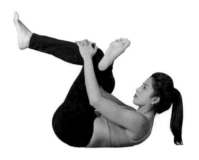

SUPINE PIRIFORMIS STRETCH

Assume a supine position. Flex the knees and rest one ankle on the opposite knee. Grasp the supporting thigh with both hands and pull it toward the chest. Hold this position for 15-20 seconds.

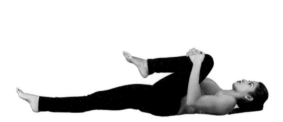

SUPINE LEG STRETCH

Assume a supine position and alternately pull each knee to the chest. Hold each position for 15-20 seconds.

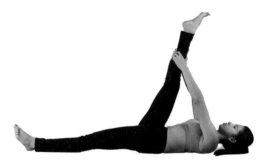

SUPINE HAMSTRING STRETCH

Assume a supine position with the legs extended. Slightly lift the shoulders off the ground and alternately pull the thigh or ankle toward the chest while maintaining the knee extension. Hold this position for 15-20 seconds.

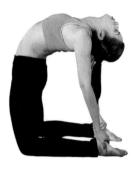

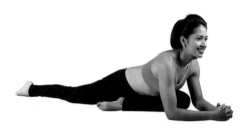

GROUNDED BACK BEND

Kneel in an upright position with the knees hip-distance apart. Gently lean backward and reach for the heels. Lift the pelvis while maintaining the back arch and elbow extension. The neck should be extended backward. Hold the position for 15-20 seconds.

GROUNDED HIP STRETCH

Adopt a lunge position and slide the rear knee back with the foot's dorsum facing down. Rest the opposite knee and both elbows on the ground with the ankle under the pelvis and lean forward to bring the chest toward the thigh. Hold this position for 15-20 seconds.

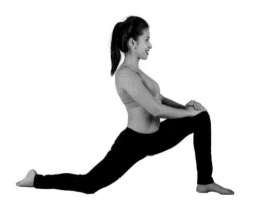

EXTENDED LUNGE STRETCH

Adopt a lunge position and slide the rear knee back with foot's dorsum facing down. Maintaining an upright torso, lean onto the front leg while supporting the hands on the knee. The front knee should not extend beyond the ankle. Hold this position for 15-20 seconds.

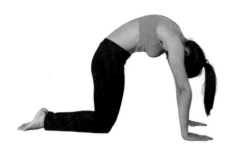 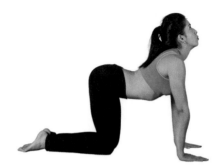

CAT AND COW STRETCH

Assume a quadruped position. For the cat stretch, arch the lower back down with neck extension. For the cow stretch, arch the back up with neck flexion, tucking the chin in toward the sternum. Hold each position for 15-20 seconds.

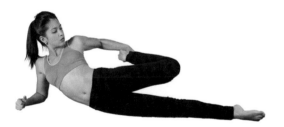 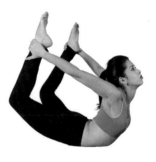

HIP FLEXORS STRETCH

Lying on your side, maintain a grounded leg extension and hold the opposite foot while flexing the knee and slightly pulling toward the glutes. Repeat on the opposite side. Hold this position for 15-20 seconds.

BOW POSE

Assume a prone position with feet hip-width apart and the arms sideways to the body. Bend the knees and extend the elbows to grasp the ankles. Lift the chest off the ground, arching the back and pulling the legs up. Hold the position for 15-20 seconds.

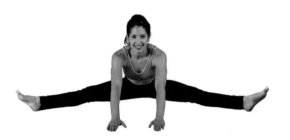

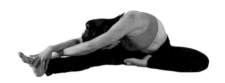

FORWARD LEAN SADDLE STRETCH

Sit comfortably on the ground with the thighs abducted and the knees extended. Maintain back alignment with the neck and gently lean forward with the arms fully extended. Hold this position for 15-20 seconds.

SIDEWAYS LEAN SADDLE STRETCH

Sit comfortably on the ground with the thighs abducted and the knees flexed. Maintain back alignment with the neck and lean sideways toward the extended leg. Gently reach for the ankle. Repeat on the opposite side, holding the position for 15-20 seconds.

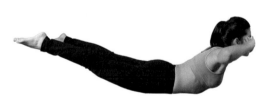

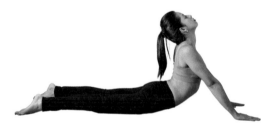

HYPEREXTENSION

Assume a prone position with feet hip-width apart and fingers slightly touching the temple. Lift the chest off the ground. Arch the back and lift the legs up in extension. Hold the position for 10-15 seconds and repeat.

LYING ABDOMINAL STRETCH

Assume a prone position. Hands should support the body, maintaining contact between the ground and the pelvis and lower legs. Raise the upper back and extend. The neck and head remain in a neutral position. Hold the position for 15-20 seconds.

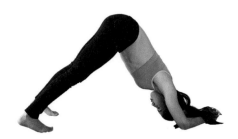 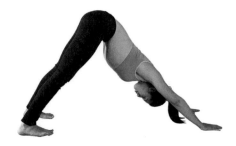

MODIFIED DOWNWARD DOG

Assume a prone position and raise the hips. Weight should be supported on the forearms with the elbows directly below the shoulders and forearms pointing forward. Fully support hipbones on the ground and allow back extension. Return to the starting position and repeat the exercise 10 to 15 times.

DOWNWARD DOG POSITION

Begin with the palms grounded and shoulder-width apart. Extend the arms and press the hips up and back, reaching the chest toward the thighs. Maintain a straight spine and keep feet hip-width apart. Heels should be fully supported on the ground. Flex the knees and lower the hips back to child pose.

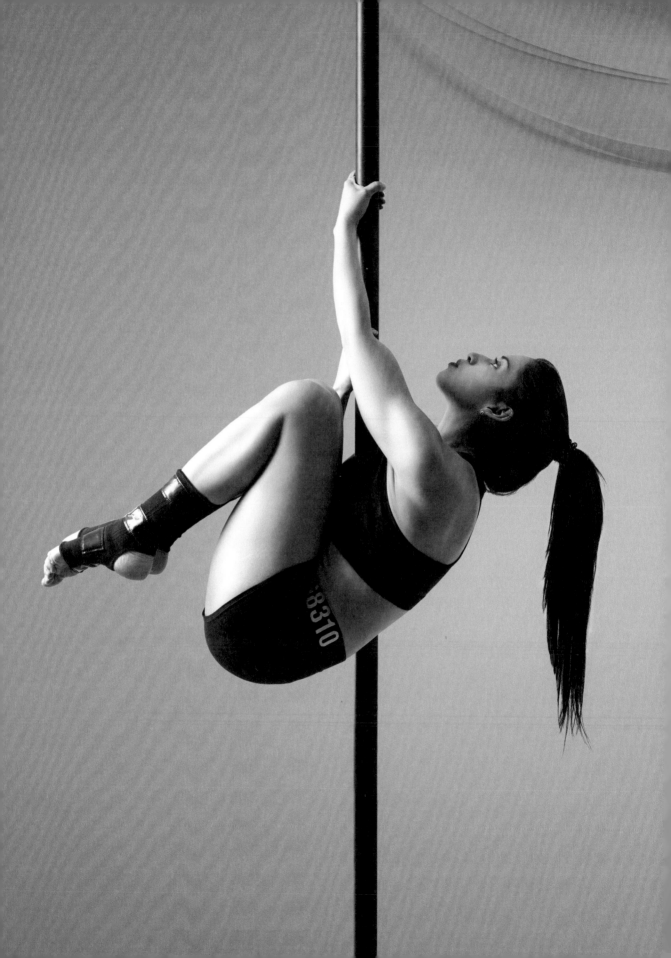

CHAPTER 3
WARM-UPS

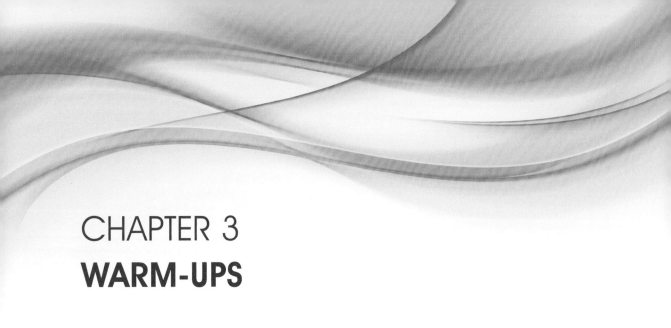

CHAPTER 3
WARM-UPS

Conditioning exercises prior to pole sessions are essential to mentally and physically prepare the body for the activities to be performed. Warm-up routines raise body temperature, increase heart and breathing rate, activate the neuromuscular system, mobilize body joints, minimize injury risks, and gradually increase resistance to prime the body for the upcoming challenges and performance improvements on the pole. Warm-up routines are recommended to achieve more effective results, and gradually increasing the intensity, number of repetitions, length of duration, and movement variations is fundamental to avoid injuries. A minimum of 10-15 repetitions on each side of the body are recommended, but it may be necessary to increase the exercise intensity to 20-30 repetitions depending on the difficulty of the supplementary workouts. Remember to warm up both the upper and lower body, focusing on the arms, abdominals, and legs.

Pole and postural conditioning exercises may be incorporated into the workout sets to complement the process, but bear in mind each challenger's capabilities and endurance. Continuous and prudent progress observation must take place in order to determine the most appropriate exercise upgrades.

INDIVIDUAL WORKOUTS

- High knee block
- Rear lunges
- Forearm plank
- Side leg lifts
- Mountain climbers
- Plank jacks

- Crab walk
- Supine bicycle
- Six-inch circles
- V balance
- Frog jumps
- Push-ups with knee support

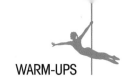

- Plank with arm lift
- Reach-ups
- Heel touch
- Backward and forward wide circles
- Plank side walk
- Basic and single-leg squats
- Extended kickbacks
- Scissors
- Bend and reach
- Standing side crunch
- Staggered hand push-ups
- Elevated crunches
- Single-leg toe reaches
- Butt kickers
- Push-ups and clap
- Reach-throughs
- Running in place
- Hip raise
- Jumping jacks
- Inchworms
- Crunches
- Cross-legged lift
- One-arm side push-up
- Front kicks
- Shoulder tap push-up
- Leg spreaders
- In and out abdominals

- Reverse crunch
- Lunge jumps
- Hip raise
- Wide arm push-ups
- Plank forearm support and lateral steps
- Six inch and hold
- Single-leg hops
- Wide squats
- Downward dog splits and pulses
- Superman exercises and swimmers
- Low-body Russian twists
- Star jumps
- Pulses and lifts
- Alternate support plank
- Single-leg push-ups
- Genie sit
- Small arm circles
- Plank side arm raised
- Hip raise and knee extension
- Scissor kicks
- Burpees
- Reverse plank and triceps dips
- Side bridge
- Plank forearm support side twists
- Jump squats
- Pike push-up

POLE WORKOUTS

- Back and forth body waves
- Body wave kicks
- Side-to-side jumps and lifts
- Switch arm pole squats
- Pole back lunges
- Front kicks
- Pole diagonal lunges
- Pole side kicks
- Windmills
- Pole push-ups
- Pole side pulls
- Oblique crunches
- Oblique crunches with pole support
- Pole squat with knees together
- Pole squat with spread legs
- Pole squat with wide legs
- Frontal pole squats (A)
- Frontal pole squats (B)
- Frontal pole squats (C)
- Grounded inversion (A)
- Grounded inversion (B)
- Seated shoulder mount (A)
- Seated shoulder mount (B)
- Seated shoulder mount (C)
- Seated shoulder mount (D)
- Backward spin and leg raises

- Tucks and lifts
- Half tucks and lifts
- Pole hold slide
- Inversion hold
- Inversion hold tucked
- Inversion hold extended
- Pole climb squat (A)
- Pole climb squat (B)
- Pole climb aerial squat (A)
- Pole climb aerial squat (B)
- Bracket grip
- Split grip full bracket (flutter feet)
- Split grip full bracket grounded knees (A)
- Split grip full bracket grounded knees (B)
- Split grip rotators
- Beginner pole climber
- Advanced pole climber
- Continuous pole climbs
- Back support tucks
- Pole hold knee flexions
- Pull-ups
- Spinning pull-ups (pencil)
- Pole chin-ups
- Layback sit-ups
- Superman push-ups
- Continuous knee hook climbs

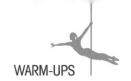

- Caterpillar push-ups

- Continuous caterpillar climbs

- Shoulder mount tucks

- Shoulder mount open V

- Iguana press

- Inverted push-ups

- One-handed handstand

- Shoulder mount bounce descent

INDIVIDUAL WORKOUTS

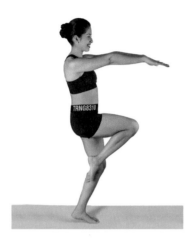

HIGH KNEE BLOCK

With both arms raised forward at shoulder level, contract the abdomen and lower both arms to the right knee. Repeat the movement on the opposite side.

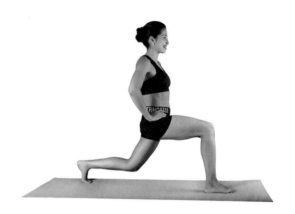

REAR LUNGES

Assume a low split position with the weight mainly supported on the front leg. Maintain torso engagement. Alternate on both sides.

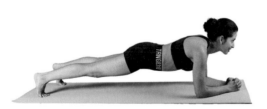

FOREARM PLANK

With the feet shoulder-width apart, support the forearms on the ground with elbows at shoulder level. Maintain contraction of abdominal muscles and glutes while ensuring body alignment. Hold position.

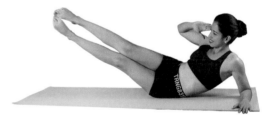

SIDE LEG LIFTS

Lie laterally on the ground with the weight supported on the elbow and ensuring body alignment. Engage the core muscles and raise legs to approximately 45 degrees and then lower them in a controlled manner.

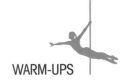

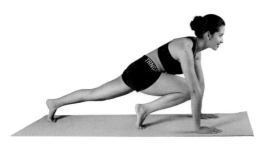

MOUNTAIN CLIMBERS

Assume a plank position with the hands and feet shoulder-width apart. Contract the glutes and abdomen. Draw one knee toward the chest and return it to the starting position. Repeat with the opposite leg.

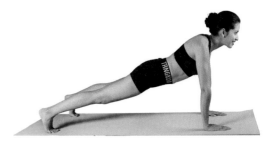

PLANK JACKS

Assume a plank position with the abdomen and glutes fully contracted. Maintain body alignment and keep the pelvis steady. Separate legs wider than hips with a slight jump and then return to the starting position.

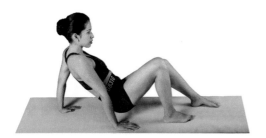

CRAB WALK

Assume a seated position. Arms are behind you, supporting the weight, and the feet are hip-distance apart. Raise the hips, engaging the abdominal muscles. Step forward, following the movement with the hands. Repeat the exercise.

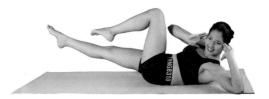

SUPINE BICYCLE

Assume a supine position and contract the abdominals while raising the head and shoulders off the ground. Rotate the torso and reach the left elbow toward the right knee with the opposite leg extended. Repeat on both sides.

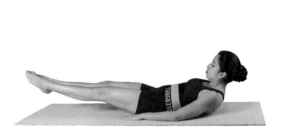

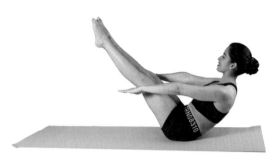

SIX-INCH CIRCLES

Assume a supine position. Extend the legs forward, maintaining ankle contact. Place the hands by the sides and slowly lift the legs approximately six inches off the ground. Hold this position, engaging the abdominal muscles. Perform a circular leg movement to the right and then repeat to the opposite direction.

V BALANCE

Contract the abdominal muscles, and raise the legs to approximately a 45-degree angle. Maintain arms at shoulder level and hold position.

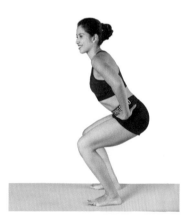

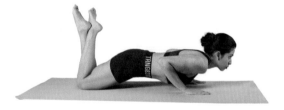

FROG JUMPS

Stand with the feet slightly wider than hip-width apart. Squat down without exceeding the knee level. From the squat position, jump up and then immediately repeat the exercise. Jump from one position to the other.

PUSH-UPS WITH KNEE SUPPORT

Assume a plank position and support the knees on the ground with ankles crossed. Bend the elbows to lower the body and push up to return to a plank position.

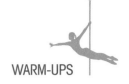

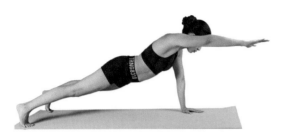

PLANK WITH ARM LIFT

Assume a plank position with the feet wider than hip-width apart. Engage the abdominal muscles and alternate raising the arms forward. Maintain horizontal plane.

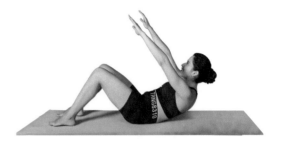

REACH-UPS

Assume a supine position. Raise the arms to shoulder level and lift the upper body off the ground, engaging abdominal muscles. Maintain back and neck extension. Lower and repeat.

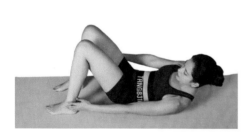

HEEL TOUCH

Assume a supine position. Lift the upper body off the ground, engaging abdominal muscles. Maintain upper-body alignment. Alternate reaching to touch the heels or ankles.

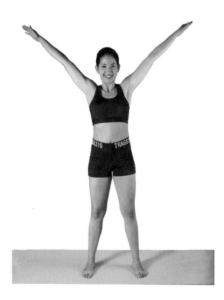

BACKWARD AND FORWARD WIDE CIRCLES

Assume an upright position with the arms by the sides and feet hip-width apart. Make large arm circles forward and backward, maintaining extended elbows at all times.

PLANK SIDE WALK

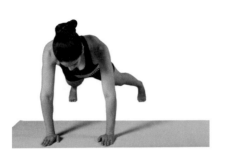

Assume a plank position with the abdomen and glutes fully contracted. Maintain body alignment and keep the pelvis steady. Separate the legs at a distance more than hip-width apart, and move sideways to the right with the right arm and leg, followed by left arm and leg. Repeat these steps to move sideways in the opposite direction.

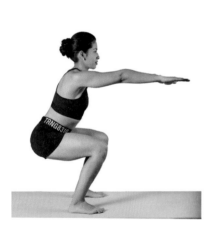

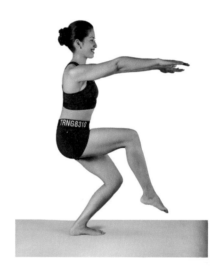

BASIC AND SINGLE-LEG SQUATS

Stand with the feet slightly wider than hip-width apart. Squat down without exceeding knee level and return to the starting position. To make it more challenging, maintain balance on one foot while flexing the knee to 90 degrees. The opposite leg remains fully extended while performing the squat. Repeat the exercise with both legs.

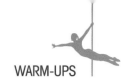

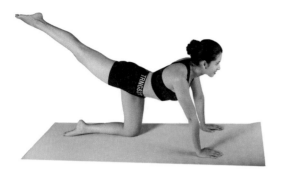

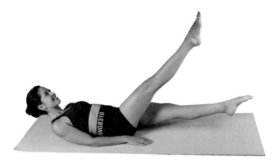

EXTENDED KICKBACKS

Assume a prone position, supporting and maintaining the knees hip-width apart. With the hands supported on the ground at shoulder level, fully extend and raise one leg backward, maintaining contracted abdominal muscles and glutes. Repeat the exercise on the opposite side.

SCISSORS

Assume a supine position. Extend the legs forward and maintain ankle contact; hands are supported by the sides. Raise the legs approximately six inches off the ground. Hold the position while engaging the abdominal muscles. Raise and lower each leg alternately.

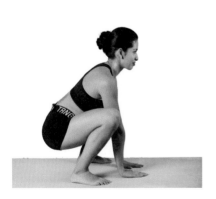

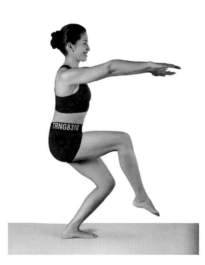

BEND AND REACH

Stand with feet slightly wider than hip-width apart. Squat down to reach the ground and return to the starting position, maintaining upper-body alignment.

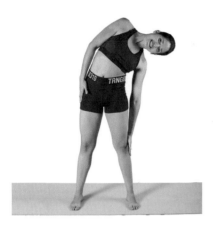

STANDING SIDE CRUNCH

Assume an upright position with the arms by the sides and feet hip-width apart. Lean toward one side, reaching with the corresponding hand to knee level. Repeat on the opposite side.

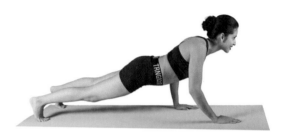

STAGGERED HAND PUSH-UPS

Assume a plank position with the hands placed in a staggered position. While maintaining body alignment, fully contract the glutes and abdominal muscles. Bend the elbows and push up to return to the starting position.

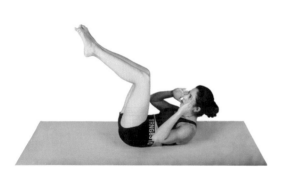

ELEVATED CRUNCHES

Assume a supine position. Lift the upper body off the ground, engaging the abdominal muscles. Raise the legs and maintain knee flexion while performing crunches. Maintain upper-body alignment.

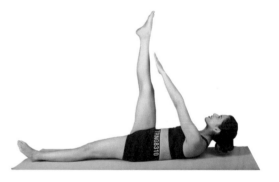

SINGLE-LEG TOE REACHES

Assume a supine position. Raise one leg to hip level, maintaining a grounded position with the opposite leg. Extended both arms fully to reach the toes. Hold the position while engaging the core muscles. Alternate raising and lowering one leg at a time.

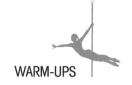

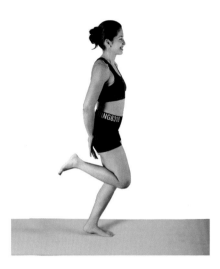

BUTT KICKERS

Begin trotting in place with a rhythmic pace. Alternately raise legs backward to gently kick the glutes.

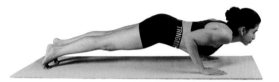

PUSH-UPS AND CLAP

Assume a plank position. Flex the elbows, maintaining contact with the body and contracting the abdominal muscles. Rapidly push up to clap hands and return to the initial position. Knees may remain on the ground.

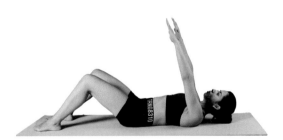

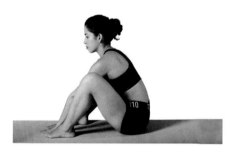

REACH-THROUGHS

Assume a seated position with the feet on the ground. Lift the upper body off the ground, engaging abdominal muscles, and reach forward between the legs.

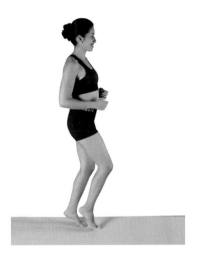

RUNNING IN PLACE

Trot in place at a rhythmic pace.

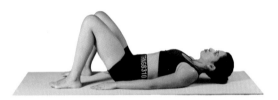 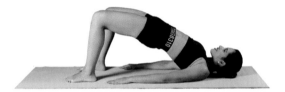

HIP RAISE

Continuously raise hips off the ground, maintaining alignment between the shoulders, back, hips, and knees. Contract the abdominal muscles, glutes, and hamstrings throughout the exercise.

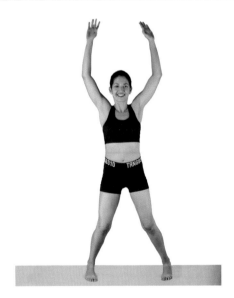

JUMPING JACKS

Begin standing in an upright position. Jump the feet farther than shoulder-width apart, simultaneously extending the arms over the head. Jump to return to the starting position.

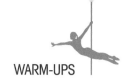

INCHWORMS

Assume a plank position with the feet wider than hip-width apart. Engage the abdominal muscles and use the fingers to walk the upper body back toward the feet. Revert the movement to return to the starting position.

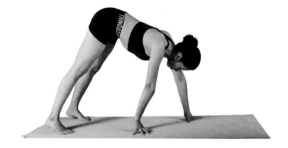

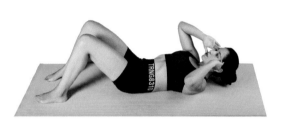

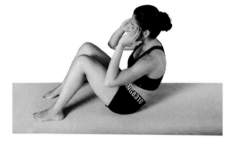

CRUNCHES

Assume a supine position. Lift the upper body off the ground, engaging the abdominal muscles. Maintain upper-body alignment while raising the chest toward the thighs with each movement.

CROSS-LEGGED LIFT

Assume a supine position with the arms to the sides. Flex one knee and cross it over the opposite thigh. Raise the extended leg to hip level and then return to the starting position while avoiding contact between the leg and the ground. The back must be fully supported. Repeat on the opposite side.

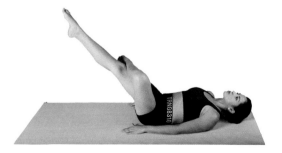

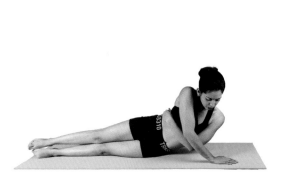

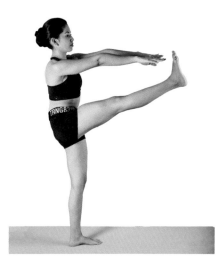

ONE-ARM SIDE PUSH-UP

Lie on the ground laterally, ensuring proper body alignment. Keep the core muscles engaged and support the far hand on the ground. Place the opposite arm on the torso and perform a single-hand push-up. Repeat on the other side.

FRONT KICKS

Assume an upright position with the arms by the sides and feet hip-width apart. Extend the arms until they are fully extended forward and then kick one leg out to touch the extended fingers. Maintain an erect back and good body alignment. Repeat on the other side.

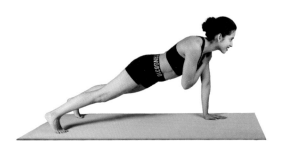

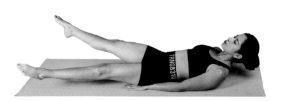

SHOULDER TAP PUSH-UP

Assume a plank position with feet wider than hip-width apart. Engage the abdominal muscles and alternate tapping the shoulders with the opposite hands. Using one hand for support, maintain stability and horizontal plane.

LEG SPREADERS

Assume a supine position with the legs extended to the front. Place the hands by the sides and slowly lift the legs until they are approximately six inches off the ground. Hold the position, engaging the abdominal muscles, and abduct both legs. Return to starting position and repeat exercise.

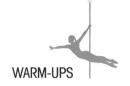
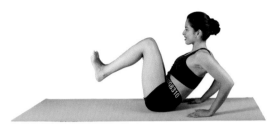 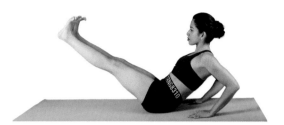

IN AND OUT ABDOMINALS

Assume a seated position. Hands should be supported on the ground with the fingers facing the hips. Elevate the legs forward, maintaining ankle contact. Engage the abdominal muscles, flex the knees toward the chest, and extend back to the starting position. Repeat exercise.

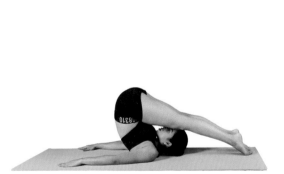 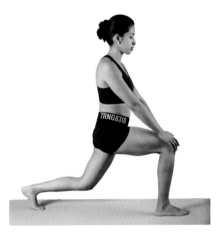

REVERSE CRUNCH

Assume a supine position. Raise both legs to hip level, maintaining contact between the ankles. Both arms should be fully extended by the sides. Invert the legs backward, engaging the abdominal muscles. Return to the starting position and repeat exercise.

LUNGE JUMPS

Assume a lunge position. Place the hands on the front knee and perform a rapid jump to switch legs, landing again in a lunge position.

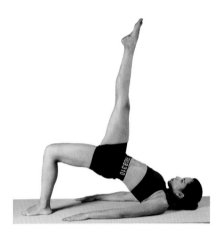

HIP RAISE (WITH EXTENDED LEG)

Raise hips off the ground, maintaining alignment between the shoulders, back, hips, and knees. Keep the abdominal muscles, glutes, and hamstrings fully contracted throughout the exercise. Raise one leg up and maintain extension while continuing to raise the hips off the ground.

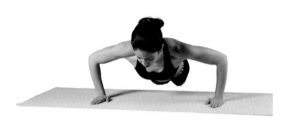

WIDE ARM PUSH-UPS

Assume a prone position, fully extending the arms and placing the hands wider than shoulder-distance apart. Legs should be fully extended and supported on flexed toes. Engage the glutes and abdominal muscles. Bend the elbows to lower the body to the ground and then push up to return to the initial position. Repeat exercise. Knees may be placed on the ground.

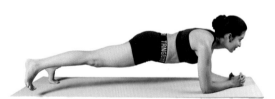

PLANK FOREARM SUPPORT AND LATERAL STEPS

With the forearms supported on the ground and elbows at shoulder level, contract the core muscles and glutes. Ensure body alignment. Take lateral steps, one foot at a time, returning to the starting position. Repeat exercise.

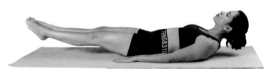

SIX INCH AND HOLD

Assume a supine position. Extend the legs forward, maintaining ankle contact. Hands should be supported by the sides. Raise the legs approximately six inches off the ground. Hold the position while engaging abdominal muscles.

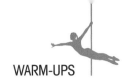

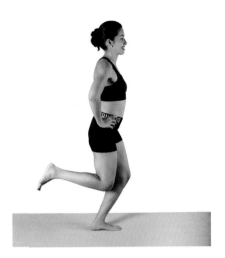

SINGLE-LEG HOPS

Assume an upright position. Flex one knee backward, maintaining stability on the opposite leg. Perform slight jumps on the supporting leg. Repeat exercise on opposite leg.

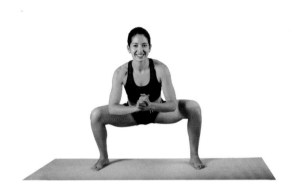

WIDE SQUATS

Stand with the feet wider than hip-width apart. Squat down until the thighs are on the horizontal plane and then return to the starting position. Maintain upper-body alignment.

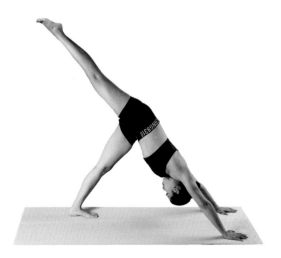

DOWNWARD DOG SPLITS AND PULSES

Comfortably place the knees on the ground directly below the hips with the hands slightly forward at shoulder level. Toes are flexed and in contact with the ground. Extend the knees, lengthening the tailbone and maintaining back and head alignment. Press the chest toward the ground as the thighs rotate outward and one leg lifts back and up, performing gentle pulses. Repeat exercise with opposite leg.

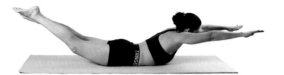 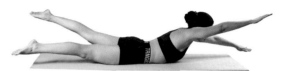

SUPERMAN EXERCISES AND SWIMMERS

Superman exercises: Assume a prone position. Arms and legs should be fully extended on the ground before being lifted up simultaneously. Keep the chest and hamstrings elevated. Hold this position for a minimum of five seconds and then repeat the exercise.

Swimmers: Assume a prone position. Arms and legs are fully extended on the ground before being lowered and raised alternately. Keep the chest and hamstrings elevated.

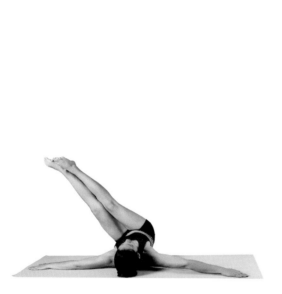

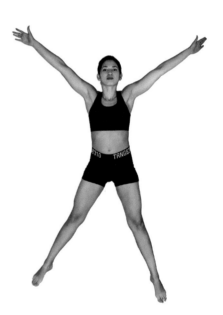

LOW-BODY RUSSIAN TWISTS

Assume a supine position with the arms fully extended sideways at shoulder level. Raise the legs to hip level, engaging the abdominal muscles engaged. Turn the waist to the right and left sides in a controlled movement. Repeat the exercise.

STAR JUMPS

Begin standing in an upright position. With the knees flexed, jump and fully extend the arms and legs simultaneously. The arms should raise sideways and the feet should be farther than shoulder-width apart. Return to the starting position.

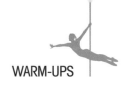

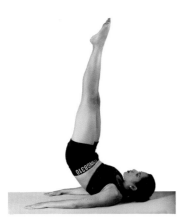

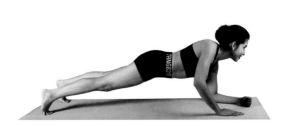

PULSES AND LIFTS

Assume a supine position. Arms are fully extended and supported sideways. Raise the legs to hip level, engage the abdominal muscles, and raise the hips and glutes, pushing toward the ground with the hands. Maintain ankle contact and keep the legs extended. Repeat the exercise, creating a pulse movement by continuously raising and lowering the hips and glutes.

ALTERNATE SUPPORT PLANK

Assume a plank position with feet shoulder-width apart and hands at shoulder level. Contract the core muscles and glutes to ensure body alignment. Alternate supporting forearms on the ground and push up to return to a plank position.

SINGLE-LEG PUSH-UPS

Assume a plank position with feet shoulder-width apart and hands at shoulder level. Contract the core muscles and glutes to ensure body alignment. Raise one leg backward and maintain the extension. Bend the elbows and push up to return to the starting position. Repeat the exercise on the opposite side.

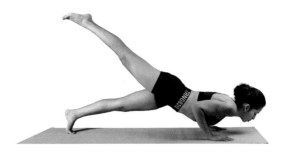

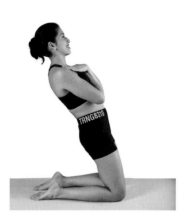

GENIE SIT

Comfortably place the knees hip-distance apart on the ground and maintain toe contact to the back. The toes should be flat under the body. Keeping the arms crossed over the chest to engage the quads, hamstrings, glutes, and abdominal muscles, moderately lean backward, ensuring back alignment. Return to the starting position and repeat the exercise.

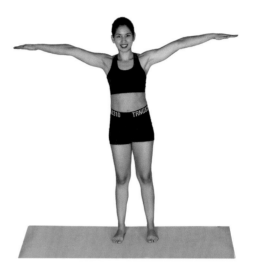

SMALL ARM CIRCLES

Assume an upright position with the arms extended sideways at shoulder level and feet hip-width apart. Perform moderate shoulder rotations forward and backward, keeping the elbows extended at all times.

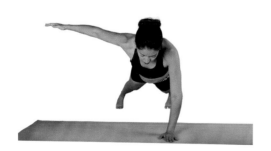

PLANK SIDE ARM RAISED

Assume a plank position with the feet wider than hip-width apart. Engage the abdominal muscles and alternate lifting the arms to the front with elbows fully extended. Maintain one-hand support, stability, and horizontal plane.

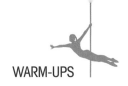

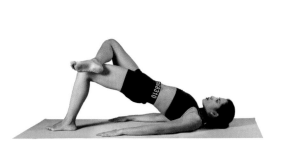

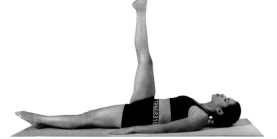

HIP RAISE AND KNEE EXTENSION

Raise the hips off the ground, maintaining alignment of the shoulders, back, hips, and knees. Keep the abdominal muscles, glutes, and hamstrings fully contracted throughout the exercise. Alternate supporting one knee over the opposite leg. Repeat the exercise, holding the position for a minimum of two seconds.

SCISSOR KICKS

Assume a supine position. Extend both arms alongside the body. Raise one leg to hip level, keeping the opposite leg approximately six inches from the ground. Engage the abdominal muscles and maintain full back support. Alternate raising and lowering one leg at a time.

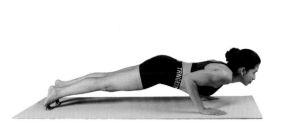

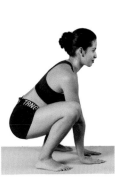

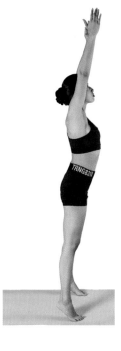

BURPEES

Stand with feet slightly wider than hip-width apart. Squat down, placing the hands on the ground and jump the feet backward into a plank position. Flex the elbows and then push up, jumping the feet toward the hands and extending the arms overhead. Return to the starting position and repeat.

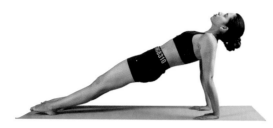 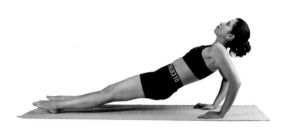

REVERSE PLANK AND TRICEPS DIPS

Reverse plank: Assume a reverse plank position with the hands and forearms supported behind you shoulder-width apart and the legs fully extended, maintaining contact between the heels and the ground. Ensure proper body alignment. Hold this position for a minimum of 15 seconds and repeat exercise.

Triceps dips: Assume a seated position with the hands supported behind you shoulder-width apart, arms fully extended, and knees flexed with feet flat on the ground. Maintaining elevated hips and glutes, flex the elbows and return to the starting position. Repeat.

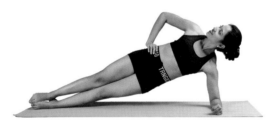 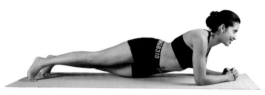

SIDE BRIDGE

Lie laterally on the ground, ensuring body alignment. Contract the glutes and abdominal muscles while supporting the forearm on the ground. Place the opposite hand on the waist. Lift the hips, ensuring proper alignment of feet, legs, back, shoulders, and neck. Return to starting position and repeat.

PLANK FOREARM SUPPORT SIDE TWISTS

Begin with the forearms supported on the ground and elbows at shoulder level, keeping the abdominal muscles and glutes contracted. Ensure proper body alignment. With the feet shoulder-width apart, twist the hips, approaching the ground from the right to the left side. Repeat.

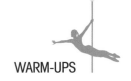

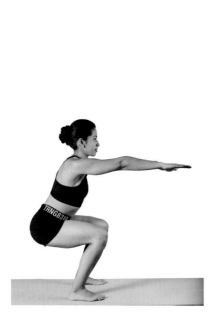

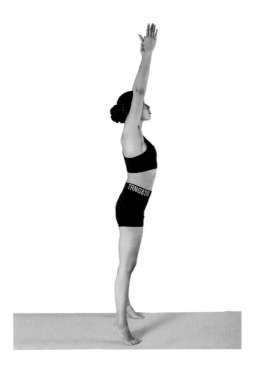

JUMP SQUATS

Stand with the feet slightly wider than hip-width apart. Squat down without exceeding knee level and jump up with the arms fully extended. Repeat.

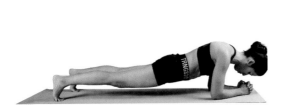

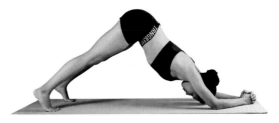

PIKE PUSH-UP

Assume a forearm-supported plank position with the feet wider than hip-width apart. Engage the abdominal muscles and bend at the hips, pressing the chest toward the extended legs. Return to the starting position and repeat.

POLE WORKOUTS

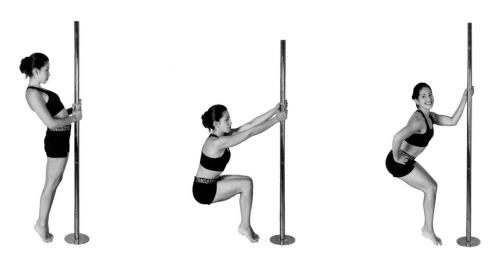

BACK AND FORTH BODY WAVES

Assume an upright position facing the pole and grasp it at chest level. Keep the feet stationary and flex the knees, bringing the chest toward the pole, then extend the knees and arch the back, simulating a full body-wave movement. Repeat exercise in reverse.

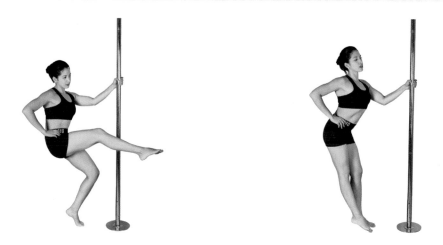

BODY WAVE KICKS

Assume an upright position facing the pole and grasp it at chest level. Keep the feet stationary and flex the knees, bringing the chest toward the pole. While the knees extend, raise either leg forward, continuing the body-wave movement. Arch the back and balance on the supporting leg. Repeat.

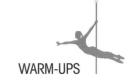

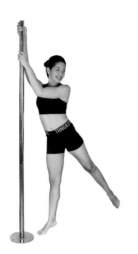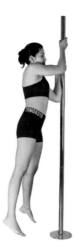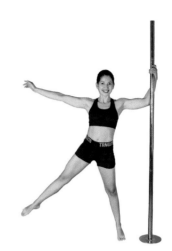

SIDE-TO-SIDE JUMPS AND LIFTS

Assume an upright position facing sideways to the pole. Grasp the pole at shoulder-level with the near hand (elbow should be flexed). Turn the body toward the pole, holding it with both hands while performing a slight jump with the knees extended. Ground the feet on the opposite side. Repeat.

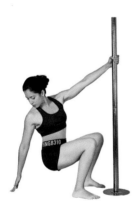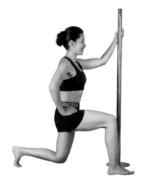

SWITCH ARM POLE SQUATS

Assume an upright position facing the pole and grasp it at chest level. Feet should be slightly wider than hip-width apart. Squat down, extending one hand backward, and return to starting position. Repeat the exercise alternating hands gripping the pole. Maintain appropriate upper-body alignment.

POLE BACK LUNGES

Assume an upright position facing sideways to the pole. The near hand holds the pole at shoulder level, maintaining a flexed elbow. The far leg takes a wide step backward, bringing the knee almost to the ground, and then returns to the starting position. Repeat exercise on both sides.

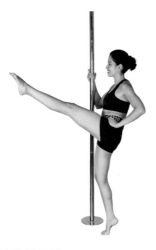

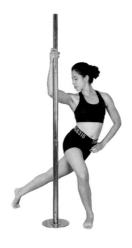

FRONT KICKS

Assume an upright position facing sideways to the pole. Raise the right leg to the front with a brushing action of the foot, engaging the gluteus, hamstring, adductor, and quad muscles. Alternate sides.

POLE DIAGONAL LUNGES

Assume an upright position facing sideways to the pole. The near hand holds the pole at shoulder level, maintaining a flexed elbow. The far leg takes a wide step diagonally backward, bringing the knee almost to the ground, and returns to the starting position. Repeat exercise on both sides.

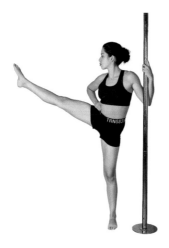

POLE SIDE KICKS

Assume an upright position facing sideways to the pole. The near hand holds the pole at shoulder level, maintaining a flexed elbow. The far leg kicks up laterally and returns to the starting position. Repeat exercise on both sides.

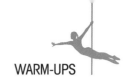

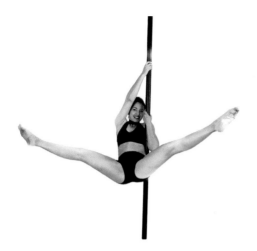

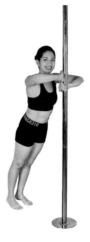

WINDMILLS

Assume an upright position facing sideways to the pole, maintaining shoulder stability and a strong hold grip. The lower body is in front of the pole. Flex the hips with extended knees and abducted thighs. Supporting the near hip on the pole, elevate first the near leg and then the far leg in a clockwise rotation. Repeat exercise in both directions.

POLE PUSH-UPS

Assume an upright position facing the pole and support both palms at chest level. Take a step away from the pole, fully extending the elbows. When confident, flex the elbows out, maintaining body alignment, and then return to the starting position. Repeat.

POLE SIDE PULLS

Assume an upright position facing sideways to the pole. The near foot should be supported on the pole. The near hand holds the pole at shoulder level, maintaining a flexed elbow and full-body alignment. When confident, fully extend the near elbow. Return to starting position. Repeat.

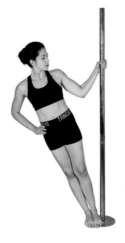

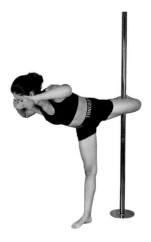 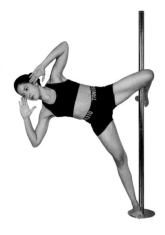

OBLIQUE CRUNCHES

Assume an upright position facing sideways to the pole. The near hand holds the pole at shoulder level, maintaining flexed elbows. When confident, hook the back of the near leg's knee around the pole, turning the trunk and chest toward the ground. Release hands from the pole. Elevate the upper body, maintaining alignment with the horizontal plane. Return to starting position. Repeat.

OBLIQUE CRUNCHES WITH POLE SUPPORT

Assume an upright position facing sideways to the pole. The near hand holds the pole at shoulder level, maintaining a flexed elbow. The far foot is supported on the pole. When confident, hook back of the near leg's knee on the pole to laterally bend the upper body and maintain alignment with the horizontal plane. Return to starting position. Repeat.

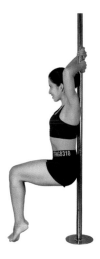

POLE SQUAT WITH KNEES TOGETHER

Comfortably support the back on the pole, maintaining adducted legs and extending the arms overhead in a cup grip. Step forward, sliding the back down the pole while maintaining flexed feet plantar. Knees and ankles should remain in alignment. Return to starting position and repeat.

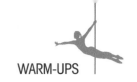

POLE SQUAT WITH SPREAD LEGS

Comfortably support the back on the pole, maintaining legs abducted slightly wider than hip-width apart and extending the arms overhead in a cup grip. Step forward, sliding the back down the pole while maintaining flexed feet plantar. Knees and ankles should remain in alignment. Return to starting position and repeat.

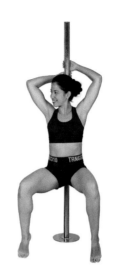

POLE SQUAT WITH WIDE LEGS

Comfortably support the back on the pole, maintaining legs abducted wider than hip-width apart and extending the arms overhead in a cup grip. Step forward, sliding the back down the pole while maintaining flexed feet plantar. Knees and ankles should remain in alignment. Return to starting position and repeat.

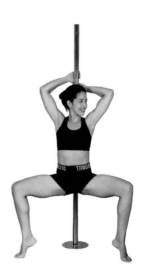

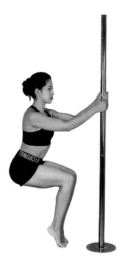

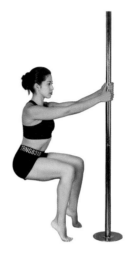

FRONTAL POLE SQUATS (A)

Assume an upright position facing the pole, maintaining adducted legs adducted and flexed feet plantar. Squat down without exceeding knee level and return to the starting position while contracting the glutes.

FRONTAL POLE SQUATS (B)

Assume an upright position facing the pole with the legs abducted slightly wider than hip-width apart and the feet plantar flexed. Squat down without exceeding knee level and then return to the starting position while contracting the glutes.

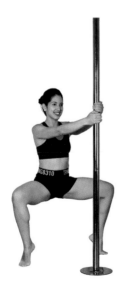

FRONTAL POLE SQUATS (C)

Assume an upright position facing the pole with the legs abducted wider than hip-width apart and the feet plantar flexed. Squat down without exceeding knee level and return to the starting position while contracting the glutes.

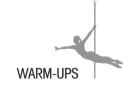

GROUNDED INVERSION (A)

Assume a supine position with the legs adducted and fully extended on the ground. Ensure a strong hold grip. Maintain back contact with the ground and bring the flexed knees toward the chest. Return to the starting position and repeat the exercise on the opposite side.

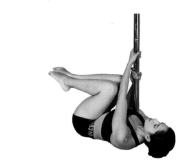

GROUNDED INVERSION (B)

Assume a supine position with the legs adducted and fully extended. Ensure a strong hold grip. When confident, raise the hips off the ground and bring them toward the chest. Abduct and extend the legs over the head to reach the ground. Return to the starting position and repeat the exercise on the opposite side.

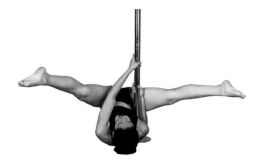

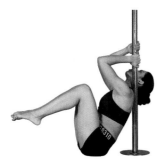 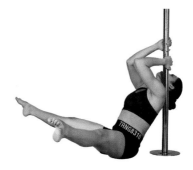

SEATED SHOULDER MOUNT (A)

Facing away from the pole, assume a comfortable seated position while maintaining upper back support between the spine and shoulder. The lower back should be far from the pole and the legs should be adducted and fully extended on the ground. Ensure an overhead cup grip and bring the flexed knees toward the chest. Return to the starting position and repeat the exercise on the opposite side.

SEATED SHOULDER MOUNT (B)

Facing away from the pole, assume a comfortable seated position while maintaining upper back support between the spine and shoulder. The lower back should be far from the pole and the legs should be abducted and fully extended on the ground. Ensure an overhead cup grip and bring the extended knees toward the chest. Return to the starting position and repeat on the opposite side.

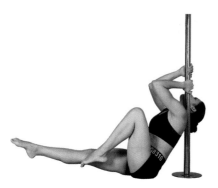

SEATED SHOULDER MOUNT (C)

Facing away from the pole, assume a comfortable seated position while maintaining upper back support between the spine and shoulder. The lower back should be distant from the pole and the legs should be slightly abducted and fully extended on the ground. Ensure an overhead cup grip and alternately bring one flexed knee toward the chest while the opposite leg remains elevated parallel to the ground. Repeat the exercise on the opposite side.

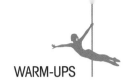
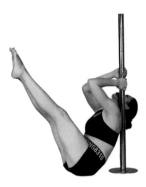

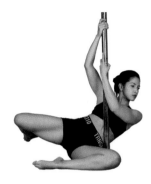

SEATED SHOULDER MOUNT (D)

Facing away from the pole, assume a comfortable seated position while maintaining upper back support between the spine and shoulder. The lower back should be distant from the pole and the legs should be together and fully extended on the ground. Ensure an overhead cup grip and bring the extended knees toward the chest. Return to the starting position and repeat on the opposite side.

BACKWARD SPIN AND LEG RAISES

Begin in the basic backwards attitude. Spin down the pole until the legs reach the ground. Remain in a grounded double attitude leg position and repeatedly raise the far leg. Return to the starting position and repeat the exercise on the opposite side.

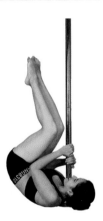

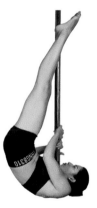

TUCKS AND LIFTS

Assume a supine position with the legs adducted and fully extended on the ground. Ensure a cup grip and shoulder mount support on pole. Maintain back contact with the ground and bring the flexed knees toward the chest. Return to the starting position and repeat the exercise on the opposite side.

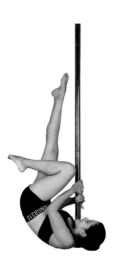

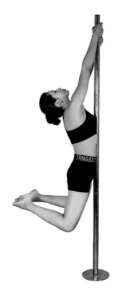

HALF TUCKS AND LIFTS

Assume a supine position with the legs adducted and fully extended on the ground. Ensure an overhead cup grip. When confident, raise the hips off the ground to alternately bring one flexed knee toward the chest while the opposite leg remains elevated parallel to the pole. Repeat the exercise, exchanging hand position.

POLE HOLD SLIDE

Assume an upright position facing the pole and grasp it above chest level with extended elbows. Flex the elbows and bring the chest to the pole while lifting the body off the ground. Both hips extend backwards and knees are apart and flexed 90 degrees. Toes should be in contact with each other. Hold this position and extend the arms, maintaining body suspension. Return to the starting position. Repeat.

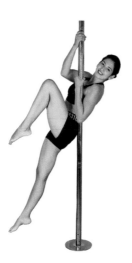

INVERSION HOLD

Assume an upright position facing sideways to the pole. Ensure a two-handed strong hold grip and hip support on the pole. When confident, engage the abdominal muscles to bring the flexed near knee toward the chest while simultaneously lifting the opposite leg slightly off the ground. Avoid jumping to perform this exercise. Return to the starting position. Repeat on the opposite side.

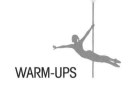

INVERSION HOLD TUCKED

Assume an upright position facing sideways to the pole. Ensure a two-handed strong hold grip and hip support on pole. When confident, engage the abdominal muscles to bring the flexed knees toward the chest. Avoid jumping to perform this exercise. Return to the starting position. Repeat on the opposite side.

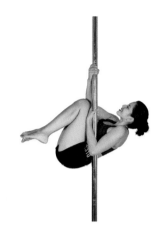

INVERSION HOLD EXTENDED

Assume an upright position facing sideways to the pole. Ensure a two-handed strong hold grip and hip support on pole. When confident, engage the abdominal muscles to bring the extended knees toward the chest. Avoid jumping to perform this exercise. Return to the starting position. Repeat on the opposite side.

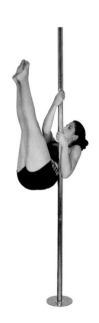

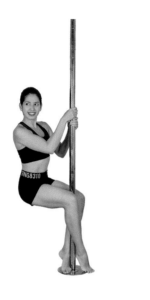

POLE CLIMB SQUAT (A)

Assume an upright position facing the pole with the legs strongly adducted, ensuring that the knees, calves, and ankles remain in contact with the pole. The feet plantar is flexed and the hands grip the pole at chest level. Squat down without exceeding knee level and return to the starting position while contracting the glutes.

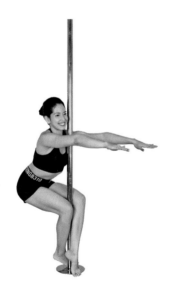

POLE CLIMB SQUAT (B)

Assume an upright position facing the pole with the legs strongly adducted, ensuring that the knees, calves, and ankles remain in contact with the pole. The feet plantar is flexed and the arms are fully extended forward. Squat down without exceeding knee level and return to the starting position while contracting the glutes.

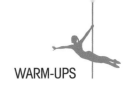

POLE CLIMB AERIAL SQUAT (A)

Assume an upright position facing the pole and grip it at chest level. Flex the knee and support the shin on the pole. When confident, lift the body, placing the opposite flexed knee to the front of the pole. Keep the legs strongly adducted, ensuring that the knees, calf, shin, and ankles remain in contact with the pole. The feet plantar is flexed. Lower the hips to the glutes and return to the starting position.

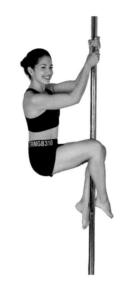

POLE CLIMB AERIAL SQUAT (B)

Assume an upright position facing the pole and grasp it at chest level. Flex the knee and support the shin on the pole. When confident, lift the body, placing the opposite flexed knee in front of the pole. Maintain strongly adducted legs, ensuring that the knees, calves, and ankles contact the pole. Feet plantar is flexed and arms are fully extended forward. Squat down without exceeding knee level and return to the starting position. Avoid resting the chest on the pole.

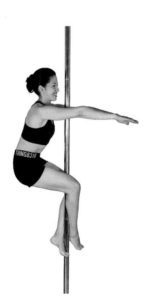

107

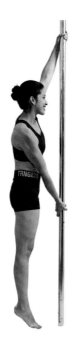

BRACKET GRIP

Assume an upright position facing the pole and ensure the pole is grasped with a two-handed full bracket split grip. The feet plantar should be flexed, maintaining contact between the feet, and the knees should be fully extended. The upper hand pulls and the lower hand pushes the pole to lift the body off the ground. Repeat the exercise, exchanging the position of the hands.

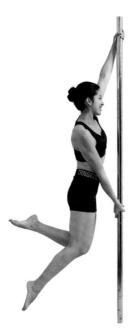

SPLIT GRIP FULL BRACKET (FLUTTER FEET)

Assume an upright position facing the pole and ensure that you are using a two-handed full bracket split grip. The feet plantar should be flexed, maintaining contact between the feet, and the knees should be fully extended. The upper hand pulls and the lower hand pushes the pole to lift the body off the ground. Hold the position and alternately flex the knees and flutter the feet. Repeat the exercise, exchanging the position of the hands.

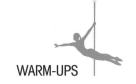

SPLIT GRIP FULL BRACKET GROUNDED KNEES (A)

Comfortably support the knees on the ground slightly wider than hip-width apart and face the pole, ensuring a two-handed full bracket split grip. The upper hand pulls and the lower hand pushes the pole to lift and slide the knees off the ground to support the flexed feet plantar. Repeat the exercise, exchanging the position of the hands.

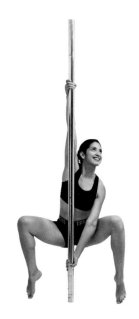

SPLIT GRIP FULL BRACKET GROUNDED KNEES (B)

Comfortably support the knees on the ground, maintaining adducted legs and facing the pole. Ensure a two-handed full bracket split grip. The upper hand pulls and the lower hand pushes the pole to lift the knees off the ground. Maintain back alignment, and the feet dorsum should be supported on the ground. Repeat the exercise, exchanging the position of the hands.

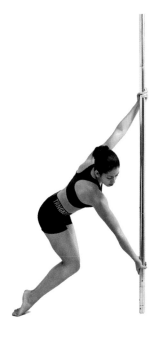

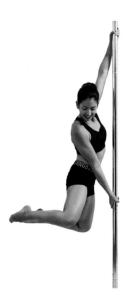 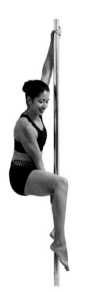 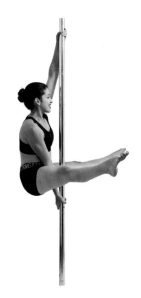

SPLIT GRIP ROTATORS

Assume an upright position facing the pole and ensure a two-handed full bracket split grip. The feet plantar should be flexed, maintaining contact between the feet, and the knees should be fully extended. The upper hand pulls and the lower hand pushes the pole to lift the body off the ground (1). Hold the position. When confident, rotate the hips forward with the knees flexed (2). Extend the knees (3) and return to the starting position. Extend both knees backward and flex to 90 degrees. Repeat exercise, exchanging hand positions.

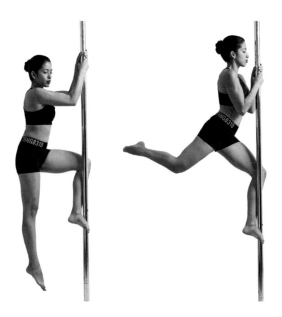

BEGINNER POLE CLIMBER

Assume an upright position and ensure that you are using a baseball grip. Flex the knee and support the shin on pole. Feet plantar and elbows should be flexed. When confident, bring the chest to the pole and lift the body (1), slightly extending the supported leg and fully extending the opposite knee backward (2). Keep the supported knee, shin, and ankle in contact with the pole. Return to the starting position and repeat the exercise, exchanging the hand grips.

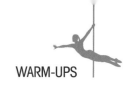

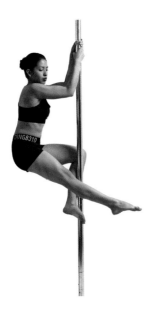

ADVANCED POLE CLIMBER

Assume an upright position and ensure that you are using a baseball grip. Flex the knee and support the shin on pole. Feet plantar and elbows should be flexed. When confident, bring the chest to the pole and lift the body, slightly extending the supported leg and fully extending the opposite knee backward. Lower the body by extending the elbows, moving the unsupported leg forward with a fully extended knee. Keep the supported knee, shin, and ankle in contact with the pole. Return to the starting position and repeat the exercise, exchanging the hand grips.

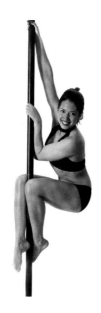

CONTINUOUS POLE CLIMBS

Assume an upright position facing the pole and ensure that you are using a forearm grip. The opposite hand grips the pole overhead with an extended elbow. Flex the knee to support the shin on the pole. Lift the body, placing the opposite flexed knee in front of the pole. Maintain forearm support and keep the legs strongly adducted, ensuring that the knees, shin, calf, and ankles remain in contact with the pole at the same level. When confident, slide the knees upwards and pull the body to exchange the forearm support. Feet plantar should be flexed. Repeat the exercise until you reach the highest level on the pole. Once this is achieved, repeat the procedure in reverse to climb down.

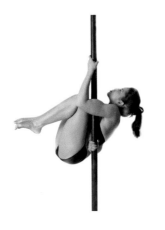

BACK SUPPORT TUCKS

Assume an upright position facing sideways to the pole. Ensure that you are using a two-handed baseball back support grip. With the back safely supported on the forearm, engage the abdominal muscles to bring the flexed knees toward the chest. Avoid jumping to perform this exercise. Return to the starting position and repeat on the opposite side.

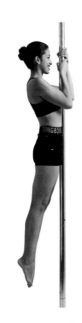

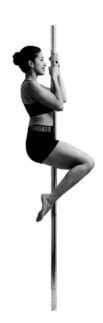

POLE HOLD KNEE FLEXIONS

Assume an upright position facing the pole and reach up to grasp it higher than chest level with extended elbows. Flex the elbows and bring the chest to the pole while lifting the body off the ground (1). Hold this position while maintaining body suspension. When confident, flex both knees up to hip level (2) and return to the starting position. The legs remain adducted. Repeat the exercise.

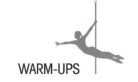

PULL-UPS

Assume an upright position facing the pole and grasp it above chest level with extended elbows. Flex the elbows to bring the chest to the pole, lifting the body off the ground. Flex the hips, abduct the thighs, and fully extend the knees. Keep the pole between the thighs and against the pubic bone, maintaining a centralized body position while climbing the pole with a hand-over-hand technique. Repeat.

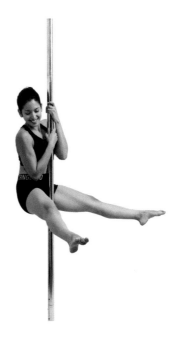

SPINNING PULL-UPS (PENCIL)

This is a variation of the pull-ups. Hold the pole higher than chest level with elbows extended and both legs extended away from the pole. Lean forward to gain momentum and, while flexing the elbows, bring the chest to the pole to lift the body off the ground. Hold this position, maintaining body suspension and leg adduction while spinning. Repeat.

POLE CHIN-UPS

Assume an upright position facing the pole and reach up to grasp it higher than chest level with extended elbows. Flex the elbows and bring the chest to the pole while lifting the body off the ground. Hold this position while maintaining body suspension and return to the starting position. The legs remain adducted. Repeat the exercise.

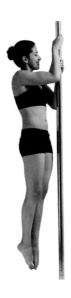

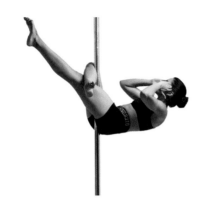 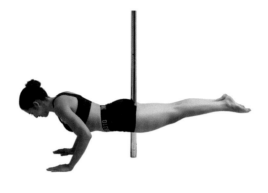

LAYBACK SIT-UPS

Begin the exercise in a crossed ankle pole sit. With the upper knee flexed and supported on the pole, hold the ankle with the opposite hand. Fully extend the opposite leg. When confident, lean back and release the hand's grip. Bring the chest toward the knees and lean back. Return to starting position. Repeat.

SUPERMAN PUSH-UPS

Begin the exercise in an inverted crucifix position. Gradually slide both legs down the pole until the hands can be supported on the ground. Flex and extend elbows, maintaining adducted thighs. Repeat.

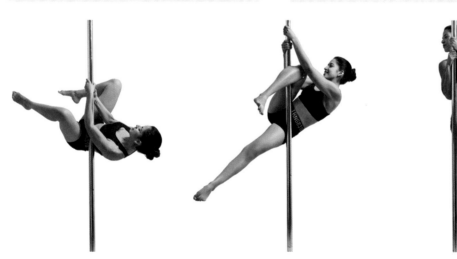

CONTINUOUS KNEE HOOK CLIMBS

Begin the exercise with body inversion. Hook the pole behind the far knee and grasp the pole above the hooked knee. Release the leg hook and extend both knees, maintaining adducted legs and remaining parallel to the pole. Strongly engage the abdominal muscles to perform an aerial inversion and continuously go over the exercise. Repeat on the opposite side.

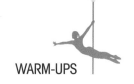

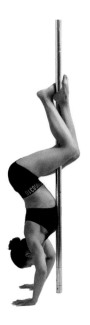

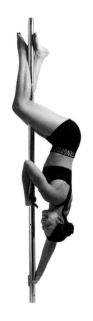

CATERPILLAR PUSH-UPS

Begin the exercise in an inverted crucifix position. Gradually slide both legs down the pole until the hands reach the ground. Elbows should remain fully extended. Support the chest on the pole and flex the knees to hip level. Maintain leg adduction. When confident, flex the elbows and extend the knees, sliding the legs on the pole. Repeat.

CONTINUOUS CATERPILLAR CLIMBS

Begin the exercise with an inverted leg hold. Ensure an inverted two-handed strong hold grip. Maintain leg adduction. Support the chest on the pole, flex the knees to hip level while pushing the body away, and extend both elbows using a two-handed half grip. Bring the bottom toward the heels. Extend the knees to slide the legs on the pole. Repeat.

SHOULDER MOUNT TUCKS

Comfortably support the shoulder (trapezius) on the pole, ensuring a two-handed cup grip. Maintain leg adduction while contracting the abdominal muscles to bring the flexed knees to the chest and hold this position. Return to the starting position and repeat on the opposite side.

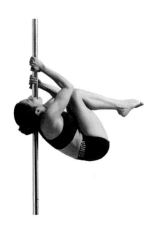

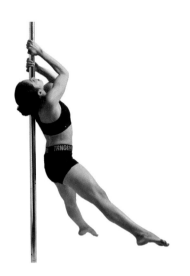

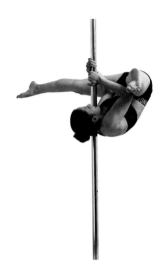

SHOULDER MOUNT OPEN V

Comfortably support the shoulder (trapezius) on the pole, ensuring a two-handed cup grip. Keep the legs extended and abducted while contracting the abdominal muscles to bring the legs toward the chest and then extend them past the head. Hold this position. Return to the starting position and repeat on the opposite side.

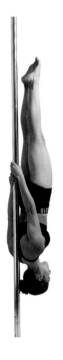

IGUANA PRESS

Assume a layback crossed-ankle position. Maintain adducted thighs and contracted glutes. Holding the pole in a two-handed iguana grip, carefully slide the body down. Maintain the leg grip. Ensure that the glutes are positioned lower than hand level, elbows are fully extended, and the upper leg foot flexion is supported on the pole for a safe grip. When confident, release the ankle grip and legs off the pole, maintaining body alignment with the legs fully adducted and separated from pole. Hold this position.

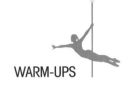

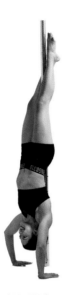

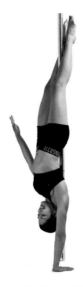

INVERTED PUSH-UPS

Assume a layback crossed-ankle position. Maintain adducted thighs and contracted glutes. Hold the pole in a two-handed iguana grip, carefully sliding body down the pole while maintaining the leg grip. Ensure that the glutes are positioned below hand level, the elbows are fully extended, and the upper leg foot flexion is supported on the pole for a safe grip. Extend the arms overhead, sliding body down to support palms on the ground. When confident, flex the elbows, sliding legs down, then extend the elbows, sliding the body up. Repeat.

ONE-HANDED HANDSTAND

Assume a layback crossed-ankle position. Maintain adducted thighs and contracted glutes. Hold the pole in a two-handed iguana grip and carefully slide the body down, maintaining the leg grip. Ensure that the glutes are positioned below hand level, elbows are fully extended, and the upper leg foot flexion is supported on the pole for a safe grip. Extend one arm overhead, sliding the body down to support the palm on the ground. Hold this position and repeat, using the opposite hand for support.

SHOULDER MOUNT BOUNCE DESCENT

Comfortably support the shoulder (trapezius) on the pole, ensuring a two-handed cup grip. Maintain extended and abducted legs and contract the abdominal muscles to bring the legs toward the chest and fully extend the knees. When confident, spring the hips up to descend, alternately lowering the hands in a hand-over-hand motion. Continuously repeat the exercise. Return to the starting position and practice on the opposite side.

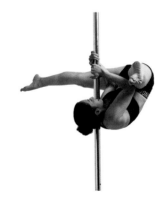

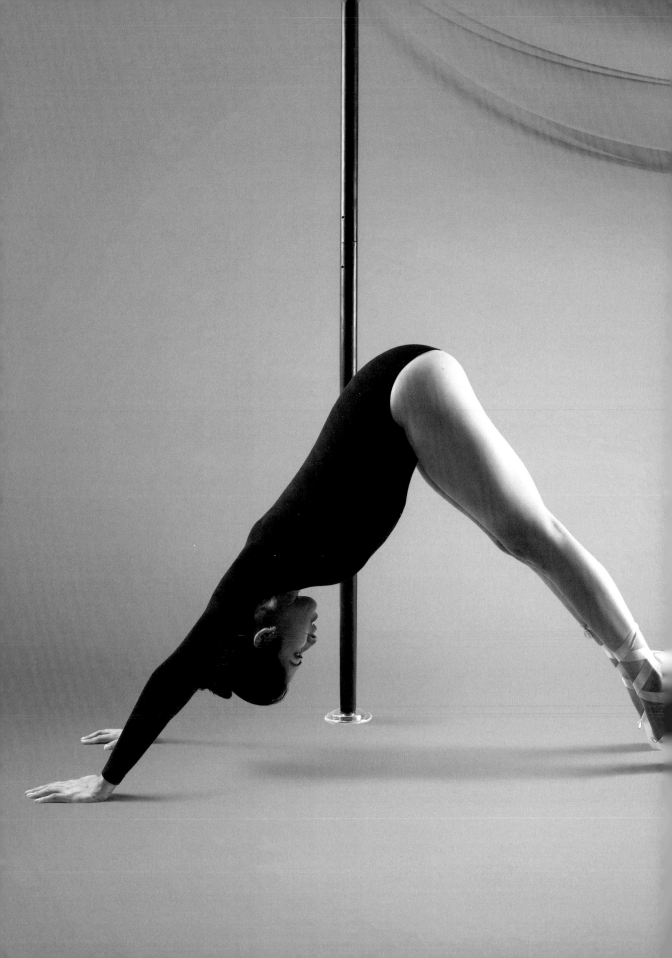

CHAPTER 4
POLE POSTURAL EXERCISES

CHAPTER 4
POLE POSTURAL EXERCISES

The main objective of postural exercises is to contribute to the body conditioning process in addition to improving posture and body alignment to optimize performance. Based on classical ballet and contemporary dance positions and movements, these exercises will significantly improve coordination, balance, and body motion control, as well as strengthening the muscles with every movement. Training the body to maintain a neutral stance and an upright position significantly minimizes injury risks, as well as preventing muscular skeletal dysfunction and arthritis. The postural chapter of this fitness guide offers readers the opportunity to select a diversity of postures and exercises according to the objectives of each workout (abdomen, arms, legs, glutes, and back). These exercise sets complement the pre-workout and must be performed cautiously and gradually, preventing overuse and excessive pressure or stress to the muscles and joints.

Challengers may choose exercises according to the tricks and movements to be performed during the pole sessions, and the number of repetitions varies according to the performer's characteristics and the quality of the exercises to be performed. A minimum of 10 to 15 repetitions on both sides of the body is recommended. To increase the exercises' intensity, 20 to 30 repetitions are suggested, depending on the difficulty of the supplementary workouts.

It is highly recommended to fully cover upper- and lower-body areas and to review the specific guidelines for a safe and effective practice.

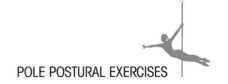

POSTURAL EXERCISES

- Neck rotations
- Alternate chest rotations
- Grand battement
- Isometric leg hold (90 degrees)
- Straddle stretch
- Knee outer circles
- Rested rond de jambe
- Isometric balanced V shape
- Forward lean
- Ninety-degree side lean (A)
- Ninety-degree side lean (B)
- Ninety-degree forward lean
- Diamond stretch
- Half butterfly pose
- Back and gluteus activation
- Camel pose

- Semi arabesque
- Anterior leg stretch
- Side grand jeté
- Relevé
- Plié relevé
- Demi plié relevé
- Rolled toes relevé
- Side port de bras
- Grand battement forward
- Port de bras forward (first position)
- Grand battement sideways
- Grand battement backward
- Port de bras backward
- Port de bras forward (second position)
- Plie relevé (first position)

POSTURAL EXCERCISES: GROUNDED

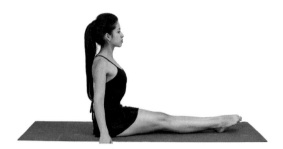

NECK ROTATIONS

Sit with an erect back, pointed feet parallel and together, and squared hips and shoulders. Gently rotate the neck and head from left to right.

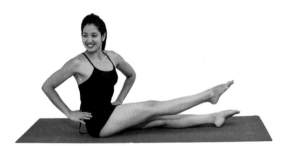 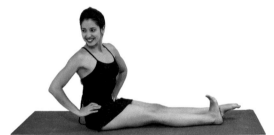

ALTERNATE CHEST ROTATIONS

With an erect back, extended legs, pointed feet, and turned-out hips, support the weight on the sit bones and place the hands on the waist. Engaging the obliques and lower obliques, keep the hips squared and rotate the torso to the right while raising the right leg. Feel the tension in the inner thighs, hamstrings, quads, and gluteus, and hold. Come back to a neutral position, dorsiflex the feet, and then rotate to the other side.

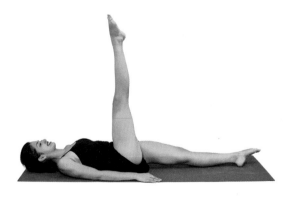

GRAND BATTEMENT

Making sure the pelvis is not tucked in, raise the leg until it is extended between 45 and 90 degrees from the hip joint using the hip flexors. Make sure you feel the length of both the working leg and the standing leg. Repeat on the other side.

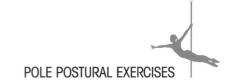

ISOMETRIC LEG HOLD (90 DEGREES)

With a flat, erect back on the floor, use the hip flexors to raise the leg and completely extend it with pointed foot turned out. Repeat on the other side.

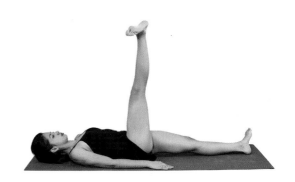

STRADDLE STRETCH

With an erect back supported on the sit bones and arms raised overhead, bend the knees while keeping the feet pointed. Slide the toes out, using the hamstrings to stretch the legs completely. Flex the back muscles and lean forward to reach a half straddle stretch pose.

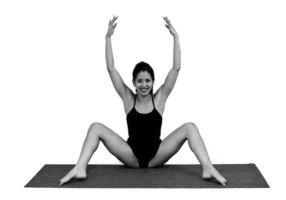

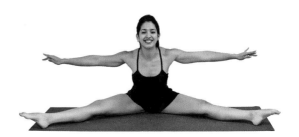

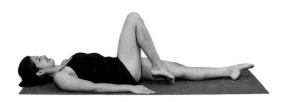

KNEE OUTER CIRCLES

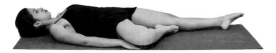

Raising a bent knee, point the feet in parallel position until the toes reach the other knee. Open the hip, taking the knee closer to the floor while continuing to engage the gluteus and hamstrings. Slide the pinky toe of the opposite foot along the floor until it reaches the other foot.

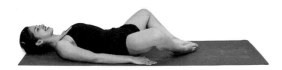

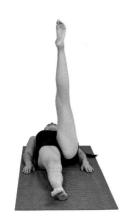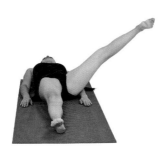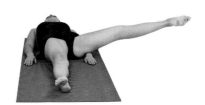

RESTED ROND DE JAMBE

With stabilized shoulders, rest on the forearms and square the hips. Perform circles with extended legs, feeling the elongation while engaging the inner thighs, hamstrings, gluteus, and quads.

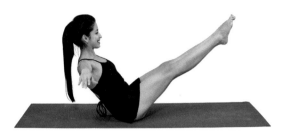

ISOMETRIC BALANCED V SHAPE

With an erect back supported on the sit bones, use the transversal abdominals and the iliopsoas to hold a 90-degree posture with straight legs. Engage the gluteus and hamstrings.

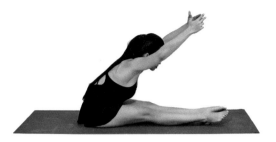

FORWARD LEAN

Extend the legs in parallel position with an elongated, erect back and arms on the same line. Feel the hamstrings stretch as you lean further forward and feel the sit bones maintain contact to the floor.

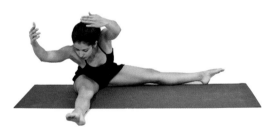

NINETY-DEGREE SIDE LEAN (A)

With an erect back and straight legs, abduct the legs from the hip joint to reach a 90-degree angle. Rotate your torso toward the right leg, making sure to maintain support on both sit bones without elevating either of them. Lean further to increase the stretch on the right hamstrings and adductors.

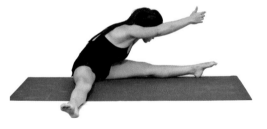

NINETY-DEGREE SIDE LEAN (B)

With an erect back and straight legs, abduct the legs from the hip joint to reach a 90-degree angle. Rotate the torso toward the left leg, making sure to maintain support on both sit bones without elevating either of them. Lean further to increase the stretch on the left hamstrings and adductors.

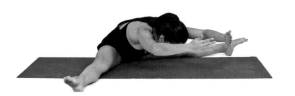

NINETY-DEGREE FORWARD LEAN

With an erect back, abduct the legs from the hip joint to reach a 90-degree angle. Lean forward, engaging the back muscles and abdominals and making sure to maintain support on both sit bones without elevating either of them. Lean further forward to feel the stretch in your hamstrings, gluteus, and adductors.

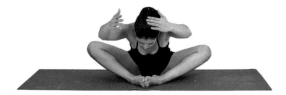

DIAMOND STRETCH

Support the erect back on the sit bones with the arms raised overhead, legs abducted, and knees bent laterally, making sure the toes touch along the midline. Lean forward toward toes to feel the stretch around the gluteal region.

Repeat the exercise leaning to the left and holding the right arm overhead with the supporting forearm on the ground. Make sure the elbow is placed underneath squared shoulders. Repeat the exercise to the opposite side.

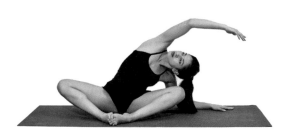

HALF BUTTERFLY POSE

From a diamond stretch position, stretch the left leg out along the line of the open hip, then tuck the right heel toward the pubic bone. Keeping the back erect, lean forward with squared hips and shoulders, stretching the right gluteus and the left adductor.

With the right hand, draw a half circle on the floor until a straight line forms between the left heel, left sit bone, and right elbow. Rest on the right forearm and lean toward the right side with an open chest to stretch the left external obliques.

Maintain hip bone support as well as squared hips and shoulders and reach both arms forward in front of the torso. Repeat the exercise to the opposite side.

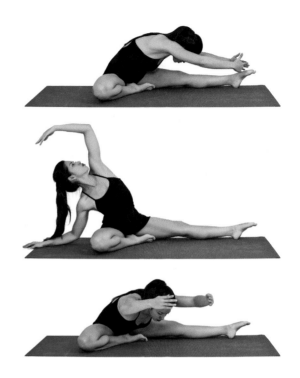

BACK AND GLUTEUS ACTIVATION

Start on all fours. The hands should be below squared shoulders, arms straight, knees below squared hips, and with an erect back. Kick pointed feet up and back with elongated legs, keeping squared shoulders and hips and arching the back while squeezing the quadratus lumborum muscle and the gluteus maximus.

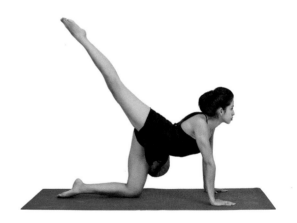

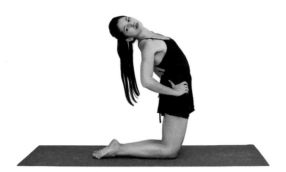

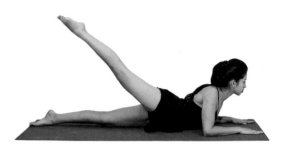

CAMEL POSE

Sit back on the knees with the feet pointed, keeping the legs hip-width apart. Lean the torso backward and hold that position while engaging core muscles but without applying pressure over the lower back.

SEMI ARABESQUE

While engaging the abdominals, the forearms lean on the ground with squared shoulders and hips, pointed feet, and straight legs. Carefully raise and hold one leg straight up as high as possible. Engage the quadratus lumborum muscle and the gluteus maximus. Alternate lifting each leg.

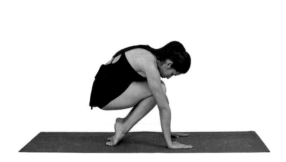

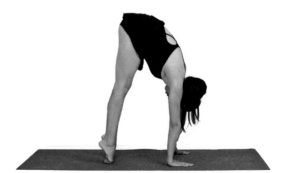

ANTERIOR LEG STRETCH

From a pronated position on the toes, support the hands on the ground. Raise the hips up as high as possible to stretch the anterior leg muscles (i.e., tibialis anterior, extensor hallucis longus, and extensor digitorum longus) and the foot arch.

SIDE GRAND JETÉ

Lie down on one side, engaging the transversal abdominals and obliques. Extend the arm of that side along the body line to support the head. The other hand should be supporting in front of the chest. From turned out hips, throw the higher leg up as high as possible, aligned with and engaging the gluteus and adductors.

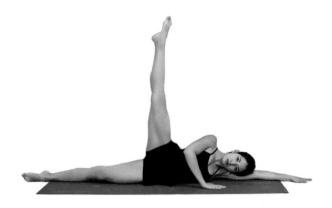

BARRE EXERCISES (ON POLE)

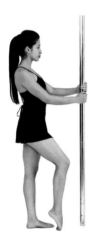

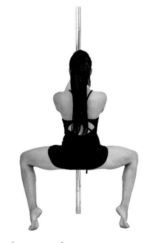

RELEVÉ

With the feet together and legs extended in a parallel position, raise one foot to demi pointe with strong legs and squared hips. Roll on the toes, stretching foot's arch, then return to parallel feet together passing through demi pointe. Alternate sides.

PLIÉ RELEVÉ

From second position with abducted hips, engage the adductor muscles and hamstrings and gradually separate the heels from the floor, contracting the gluteus and allowing the hips to abduct further as you assume relevé in second position. Engaging all previously mentioned muscles, attempt to perform a plié while abducting the hips.

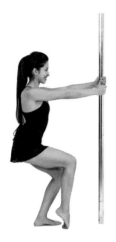

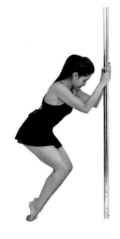

DEMI PLIÉ RELEVÉ

From demi plié position with the feet together in parallel position, alternate raising the feet to relevé. Then roll on the toes to go back to a flat-footed position.

ROLLED TOES RELEVÉ

Maintaining heel contact, relevé on rolled toes and sink low with your hips to stretch the anterior leg muscles.

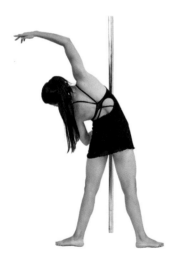

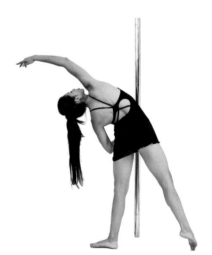

SIDE PORT DE BRAS

With the feet and arms in second position, lean to the left side while maintaining squared hips and shoulders. Raise the right arm overhead without exceeding the central line, and lower the left arm in front of the pubic bone to stretch the left obliques. Then extend the right leg and point the toes. Alternate sides.

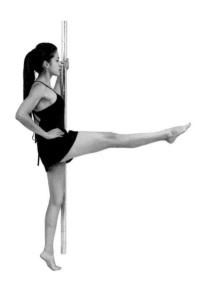

GRAND BATTEMENT FORWARD

From first position, raise the right leg to the front with a brushing action of the foot on the ground. Engage the gluteus, hamstring, adductor, and quad muscles. Alternate sides.

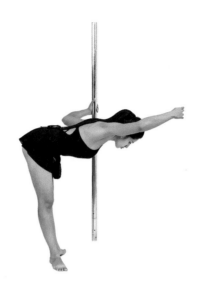

PORT DE BRAS FORWARD (FIRST POSITION)

From first position, strongly adduct the legs while maintaining an upright position and arms overhead. Lean forward, stretching the hamstrings and adductors.

GRAND BATTEMENT SIDEWAYS

From first position, raise the right leg sideways with a brushing action of the foot on the ground. Engage the gluteus, hamstring, adductor, and quad muscles. Alternate sides.

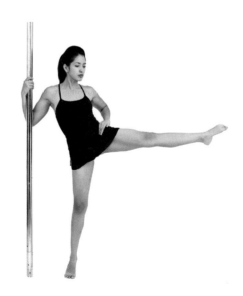

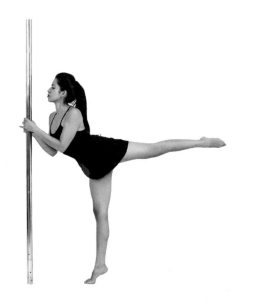

GRAND BATTEMENT BACKWARD

From first position, raise the left leg backward with a brushing action of the foot on the ground. Engage the quadratus lumborum muscle (lower back).

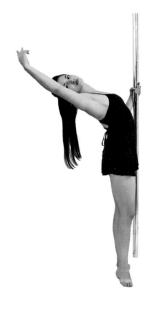

PORT DE BRAS BACKWARD

Isolating the torso, chest, and shoulders, lean backward and stretch the abdominal muscles.

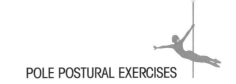

PORT DE BRAS FORWARD (SECOND POSITION)

From second position, lean forward and stretch the gluteus, hamstrings, and adductors. Avoid arching the back.

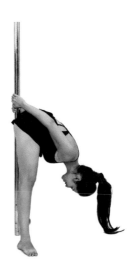

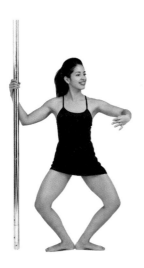

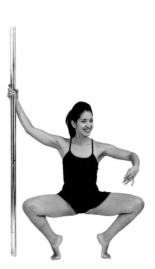

PLIÉ RELEVÉ (FIRST POSITION)

From first position, adduct the legs while engaging the gluteus, hamstrings, adductors, and quads. Lower the hips, flexing the knees outward to a demi plié. Abduct the hips, aligning the toes with the knees.

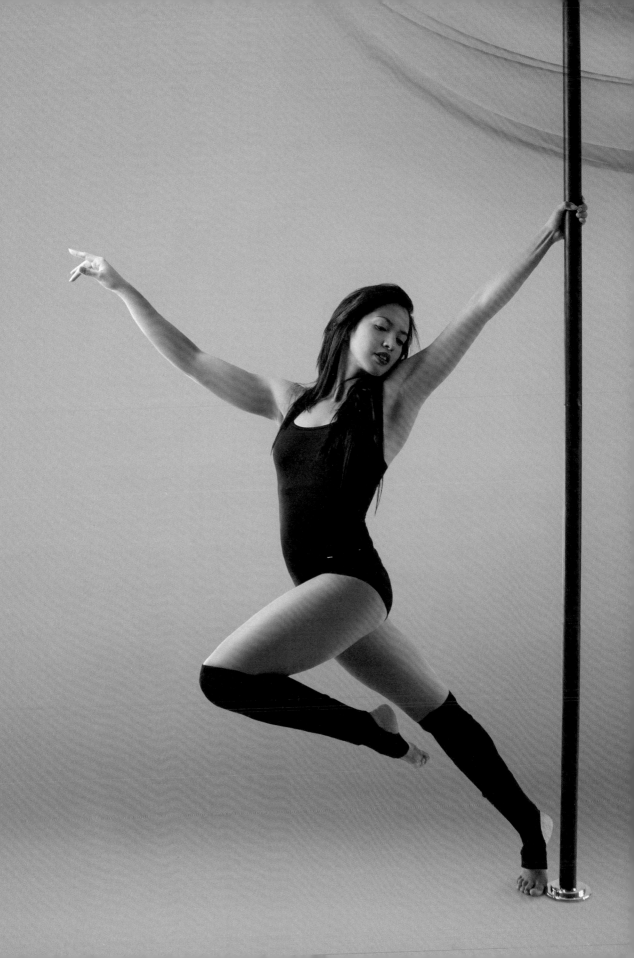

CHAPTER 5
TRANSITIONAL MOVEMENTS

CHAPTER 5
TRANSITIONAL MOVEMENTS

Transitions are an important part of pole dance performance. There are many transitional movements that may be performed, as well as improvised moves which can be combined and freely incorporated into a routine with different levels of motion complexity and speed variations. Transitions always connect to one another to accomplish a subsequent movement, spin, or stunt. A visually appealing routine places as much importance on the transitional moves as on the stunts performed on the pole. Some of these transitional moves are mainly supported on the pole, while others may actually take place on the ground, commonly known as floor work. This chapter offers a variety of movements to complement and connect with the choreography, embracing the challenger's artistic expression.

In order to create an ideal pole dance routine, it is recommended to select the pole stunts to be performed and then, once they are comfortably executed and achieved, to select the transitional movements that adapt to the various parts of the routine. It is necessary to evaluate the body position at the end of a trick in order to select and evaluate the most suitable subsequent transitions and possible additional stunts. It is important to consider the use of both the right and left sides of the body according to the stunt's qualities and characteristics, as well as the most reliable use of each side to perform each transition and trick. The guidance of a pole dance instructor may be required to assist in and contribute to the creation of an effective routine by providing useful recommendations to achieve the expected outcomes. Online sources provide an extensive selection and various demonstrations of graceful pole dance and acrobatic routines for use as creative transitional movements.

The realization of these movements requires as much flexibility, strength, and endurance as the other exercises presented. A full-body stretch and warm-up is highly recommended before attempting the provided movements. Performing a sequence of transitional movements can also serve as an effective warm-up exercise, requiring as much caution as other physical exercises in this pole dance and fitness guide.

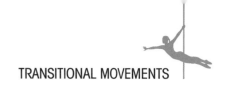

TRANSITIONAL MOVEMENTS

- Basic grip walk
- Pole peek
- Body wave
- Body wave (kick)
- Eternal pole walk
- Pirouette
- Step behind
- Reverse high hand pirouette
- Step forward turn
- Forward fold
- Pole caress
- Fairy walk
- Dip to wrap around
- Ballet hook

- Side hop
- Backslide (A)
- Backslide (B)
- Spring and slide
- Grounded wave
- Cat/panther crawl
- Floor inversion (A)
- Grounded back arch
- Grounded fan cartwheel
- Grounded star
- Floor roll
- Floor inversion (B)
- Backward floor roll

TRANSITIONAL MOVEMENTS

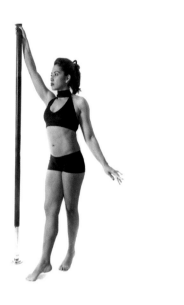

BASIC GRIP WALK

Maintain flexed feet plantar throughout the exercise. Using a one-hand basic grip, maintain an upright posture and shoulder stability while walking around the pole. Flex the knees toward the back or slide the toes with every step. To change direction, the far leg comes near the pole and the body rotates as the grip changes to the other hand.

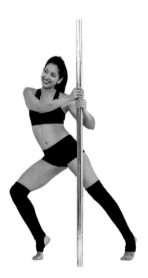 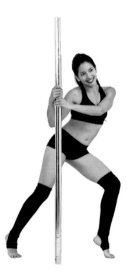

POLE PEEK

Assume an upright position facing the pole with the feet apart. Shift the trunk from the right to left side of the pole. Maintain moderate knee flexion and flexed feet plantar while twisting the toes on the ground.

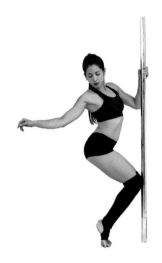 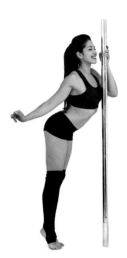

BODY WAVE

Assume an upright position facing the pole and hold the pole at chest level. Keep the feet planted and the knees flexed while bringing the chest toward the pole. Extend the knees and arch the back, simulating a full-body wave movement. Repeat in reverse.

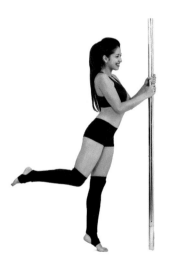 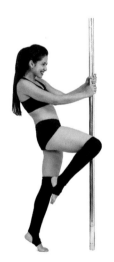 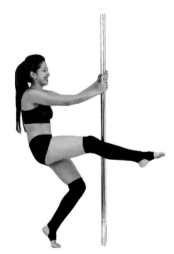

BODY WAVE (KICK)

Assume an upright position facing the pole and hold the pole at chest level. Keep the feet planted and the knees flexed while bringing the chest toward the pole. While the knees extend, raise either leg forward and continue the body wave movement. Ensure the back is arched and balance on the supporting leg. Repeat.

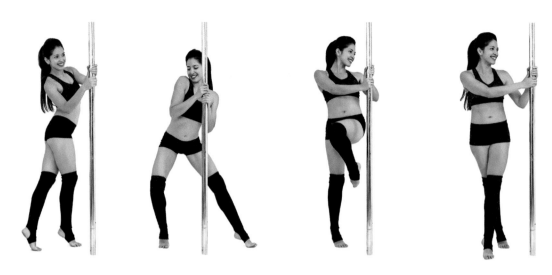

ETERNAL POLE WALK

Assume an upright position facing the pole; feet plantar should be flexed. Grasp the pole with a baseball grip. Stand with the feet apart, alternately shifting the hips and crossing the feet. Repeat.

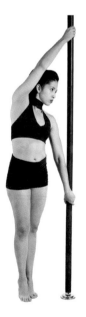 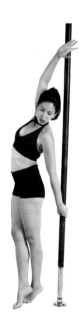

PIROUETTE

Points of support: Hands

Main focus: Maintain feet plantar flexed throughout the exercise. Focus on keeping an upright posture and stable shoulders while walking around the pole. Face the pole and grasp it using a two-handed twisted grip. Flip the upper hand, ensuring that the knuckles remain in contact with the pole. Twist on the balls of the feet, turning the body so that the head passes under the upper arm, and release the lower grip to continue the pole walk.

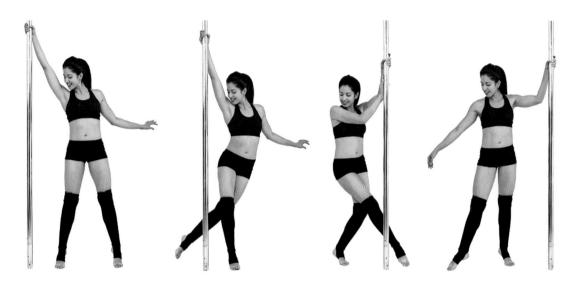

STEP BEHIND

Points of support: Hands

Main focus: Assume a body position facing sideways to the pole, maintaining an upright posture and shoulder stability. Take a side step at the back of the pole, momentarily crossing the legs, and assume the starting position on the opposite side of the pole. Maintain feet plantar flexed throughout the exercise.

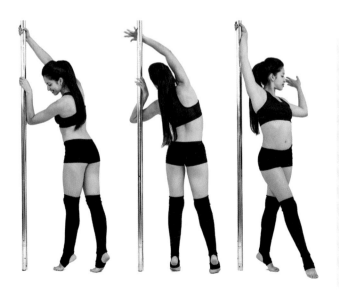

REVERSE HIGH HAND PIROUETTE

Points of support: Hands

Main focus: Maintain feet plantar flexed throughout the exercise, along with an upright posture and shoulder stability while walking around the pole. Face the pole and grasp it, using a two-handed half grip. Flip the upper hand, ensuring that the knuckles remain in contact with the pole. Twist the balls of the feet on the ground, turning the body to pass the head under the upper arm, and release the lower grip to continue the pole walk.

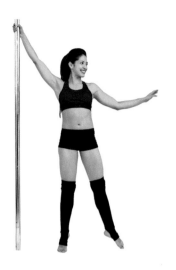 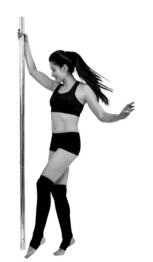 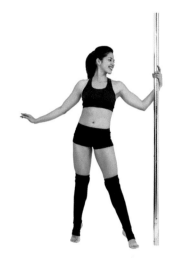

STEP FORWARD TURN

Points of support: Hands

Main focus: Assume a body position facing sideways to the pole, maintaining an upright posture and shoulder stability. Take a step forward, turning the body while exchanging the hand grip, and assume the starting position on the opposite side of the pole. Maintain feet plantar flexed throughout the exercise.

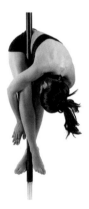
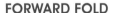

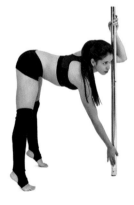

FORWARD FOLD

Stand in an upright position with the feet apart and the back supported by the pole. Lean forward, extending the arm backward (shoulder internally rotated) and keeping the tailbone in contact with the pole.

POLE CARESS

Assume an upright position facing the pole. With the feet apart and plantar flexed, lean forward and slide one hand up and down the pole. The opposite hand remains in a fixed position.

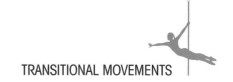

FAIRY WALK

Assume an upright position facing sideways to the pole with a one-hand basic grip. Take smooth steps while maintaining body suspension for brief seconds.

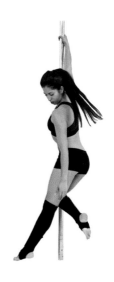

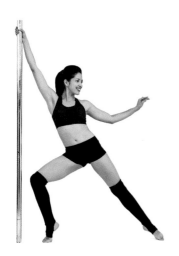 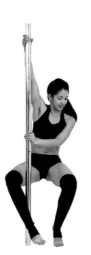 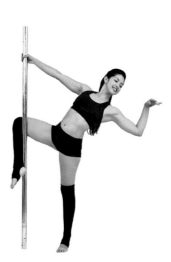

DIP TO WRAP AROUND

Points of support: Hands

Main focus: Hold the pole with a split grip and rotate the far leg forward in a clockwise motion on the ground to reach the opposite foot. Push away from the pole with a lower hand grip and hook around the pole near the back of knee while maintaining calf contact with the pole.

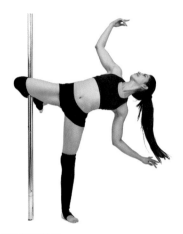

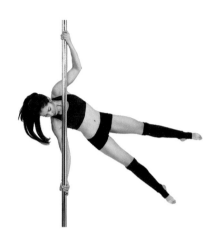

BALLET HOOK

Assume an upright position facing sideways to the pole with a one-hand basic grip. With the opposite leg fully extended, parallel to the pole, and supported on the ground, lean sideways to hook the back of the near knee on the pole and release the hand grip.

SIDE HOP

Assume an upright position facing sideways to the pole with a two-handed full bracket split grip. Raise the legs in abduction sideways to the pole and rapidly strike the ankles together in the air.

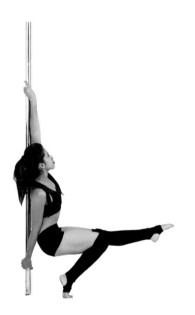

BACKSLIDE (A)

Stand in an upright position with the feet apart and the back supported by the pole. Grip the pole with a two-handed reverse grab grip. Flex the leg while gradually sliding the body down. The opposite leg remains fully extended forward. Maintain feet plantar flexed throughout the exercise.

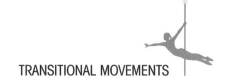

BACKSLIDE (B)

Standing in an upright position with the legs adducted and the back supported by the pole, grasp the pole with a two-handed reverse grab grip. Take the leg forward and rotate diagonally into a C shape. The opposite leg repeats the sequence. Gradually slide the body down, maintain a right angle in the hips at knee level. Feet remain plantar flexed throughout the exercise.

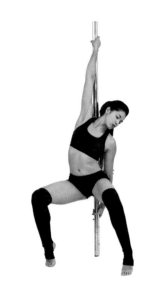

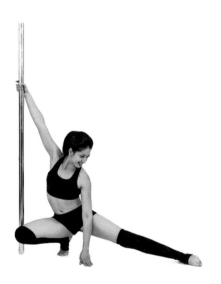

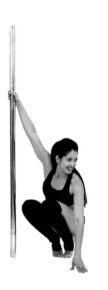

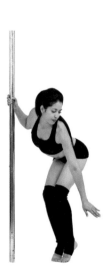

SPRING AND SLIDE

Support the body weight on a flexed knee in contact with the ground. The opposite leg remains laterally extended. Support the palms on the ground to spring the body up, bringing the legs together, and stand.

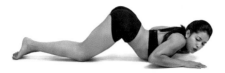

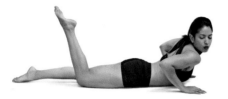

GROUNDED WAVE

Assume a quadruped position, supporting the hands and knees on the ground. Flex the elbows to bring the chest and chin to the ground. Maintain an arched back with the hips slightly flexed. Lower the pelvis while raising the upper body and extending the elbows, ensuring back extension. Repeat.

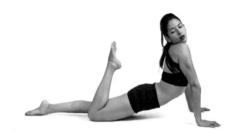

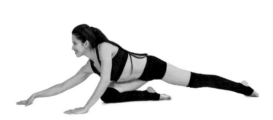

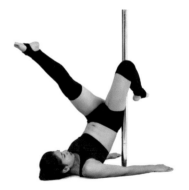

CAT/PANTHER CRAWL

Begin the exercise with one knee supported on the ground and the opposite leg extended. Lean the trunk forward, supporting the palms on the ground to crawl while alternately sliding the shins on the ground.

FLOOR INVERSION (A)

Assume a supine position on the ground. Support the arms at the side near the thighs. Raise the pelvis and fully extend the knees upward. Hook the pole with the back of the near knee followed by the opposite knee. Release the hook grip and return to the starting position.

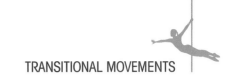

GROUNDED BACK ARCH

Assume a supine position on the ground.
Support arms at the side and arch the back
while flexing either knee toward the chest.

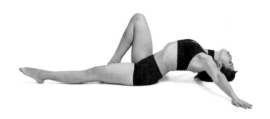

GROUNDED FAN CARTWHEEL

Sit comfortably on the ground. Lean back,
using the hands for support and raise one
leg up to rotate in a clockwise motion,
followed by the opposite leg.

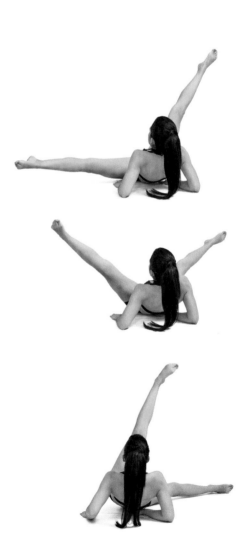

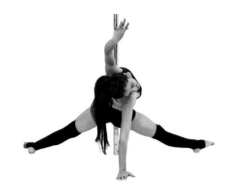

GROUNDED STAR

Sit comfortably on the ground facing the pole with the legs abducted and one arm fully extended backward and supporting the palm on the ground. Extend the opposite arm toward the ceiling. Raise the pelvis, slightly rotating the trunk sideways and maintaining heel support.

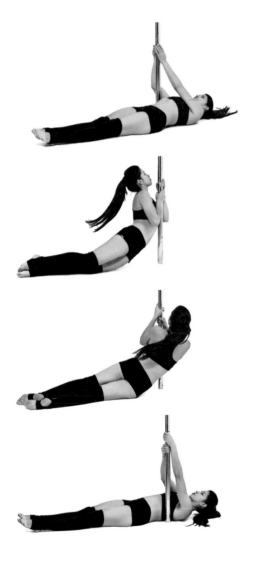

FLOOR ROLL

Assume a supine position on the ground facing sideways to the pole and using a baseball grip. Raise the upper body off the ground, turning the chest toward the pole, and roll to the opposite side of the pole. Maintain proper body alignment throughout the exercise.

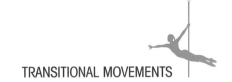

FLOOR INVERSION (B)

Assume a supine position on the ground facing sideways to the pole. Hold the pole with the near hand while raising legs, pelvis, and lower back to maintain a centralized position and the legs parallel to the pole. Be sure to use a two-handed grip.

BACKWARD FLOOR ROLL

Assume a supine position on the ground. Raise fully extended legs and pelvis off the ground to roll backwards. One arm remains fully extended while the opposite hand is supported on the ground over the head with the elbow flexed to maintain balance.

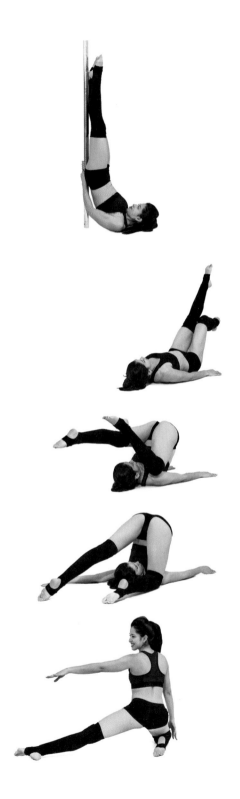

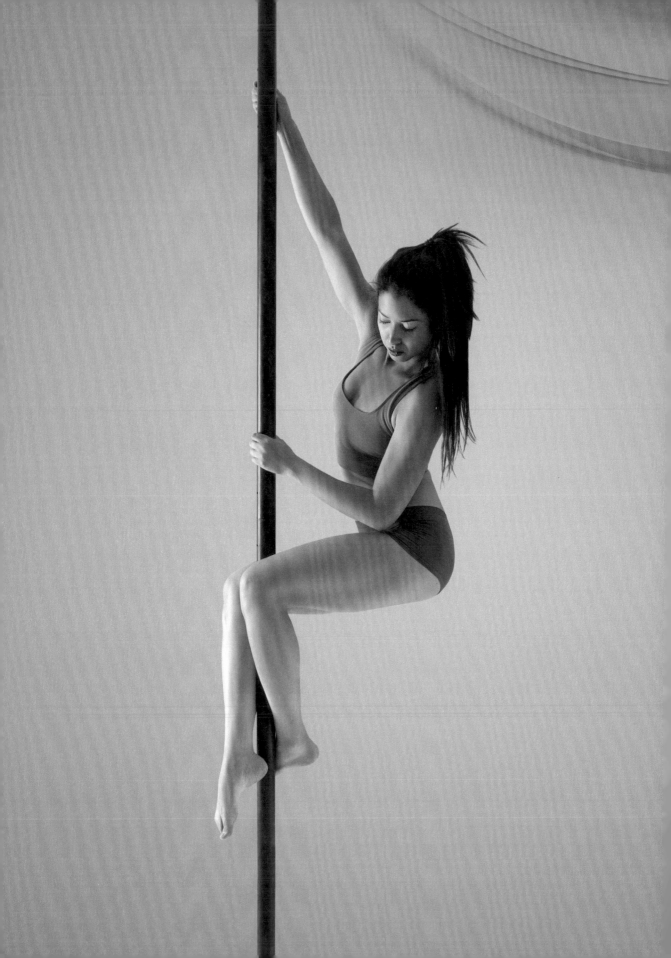

CHAPTER 6
CLIMBS

CHAPTER 6
CLIMBS

This chapter is fundamental to the performance of most stunts. The execution of many aerial tricks involves reaching higher levels on the pole by performing a variety of escalations, and climbs also serve as transitional movements between stunts. As with every trick and movement, there are varying levels of complexity when it comes to climbs. The main purpose of this chapter is to provide readers with a progressive and methodical presentation of pole climbs from the most basic to the most complex, as well as to consider the technical guidelines and to achieve a more effective and safe performance. Many pole dance tricks may be executed with equal climbs; challengers may combine and select climbs according to their routine's characteristics and genre, the demands of the stunts to be performed, and body grip reliability. Strength is continuously applied in these exercises, gradually increasing the challenger's abilities to control and fluently execute the actions. Performing continuous climbs also serves as an effective warm-up exercise to increase strength. Climbs require the same amount of caution as the other physical exercises in this pole dance and fitness guide. A review of the chapter on positions and pole principles is highly recommended before incorporating these exercises into the pole dance routines.

CLIMBS

- Basic climb
- Forearm climb
- Side climb
- Side climb variation
- Chinese climb
- Seated climb
- Pull-up climb
- Caterpillar climb
- Continuous knee hook climb

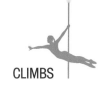

CLIMBS

BASIC CLIMB

Assume an upright position facing the pole and grasp the pole at chest level using a baseball grip. Flex the knee and support the shin on the pole. When confident, lift the body, placing the opposite flexed knee to the front of the pole. Maintain strongly adducted legs, ensuring that the knees, calf, shin, and ankles remain in contact with the pole. Pull the upper body and slide the legs upward. Repeat. Feet plantar should be flexed and posture should be upright throughout the exercise.

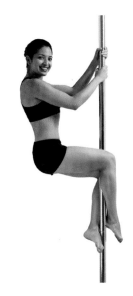

FOREARM CLIMB

Assume an upright position facing the pole. Grip the pole above your head with a forearm grip. Flex the knee and support the shin on the pole. When confident, lift the body, placing the opposite flexed knee to the front of the pole. Maintain strongly adducted legs, ensuring that the knees, calf, shin, and ankles remain in contact with the pole. Pull with the upper hand and push with the forearm to lift the body up. Flex the hips and slide the legs upward. Repeat, alternating hand grip. Feet plantar should flexed and posture should be upright throughout the exercise.

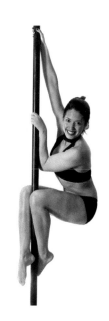

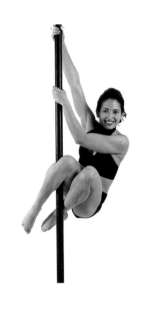

SIDE CLIMB

Assume an upright position, facing sideways to the pole and grasp it using a baseball grip. Hook the near knee on the pole at hip level. Support the anterior part of the far ankle on the back of the pole. When confident, pull the body upward, extending the legs. Take a higher grip and flex the knees to slide the legs upward. Repeat. Feet plantar should be flexed and posture should be upright throughout the exercise.

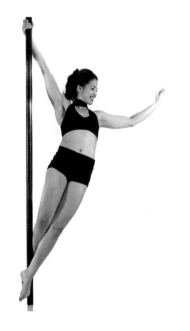

SIDE CLIMB VARIATION

Assume an upright position facing sideways to the pole and grasp it using a two-handed half grip. The far ankle is supported to the front of the pole, simultaneously supporting the anterior part of the near ankle on the back of the pole.

When confident, pull the body upward while extending legs. Take a higher grip and flex the knees to slide the legs upward. Repeat. Feet plantar should be flexed and posture should be upright throughout the exercise.

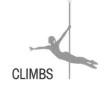

CHINESE CLIMB

Assume an upright position facing the pole and grasp it using a baseball grip with elbows extended overhead. Flex the knee and support the ball of the foot on the pole. When confident, pull the body up, supporting the opposite foot and alternating the hand grip while simultaneously taking steps up the pole. Repeat.

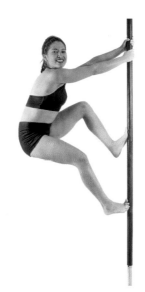

SEATED CLIMB

Assume an upright position facing the pole and grasp it using a baseball grip. The knees should be flexed at the hip and the thighs should be adducted and strongly pressed against the pole. Cross the knees to secure a thigh hold. Extend the elbows, holding the pole at a higher level, and release the thigh grip. Flex the elbows to pull body upward and adduct the thighs with crossed legs. Repeat.

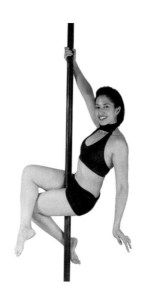

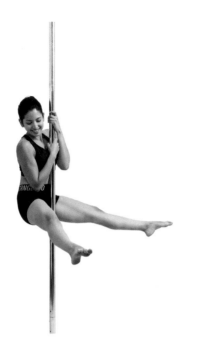

PULL-UP CLIMB

Assume an upright position facing the pole and grasp it above chest level with extended elbows. Flex the elbows and bring the chest to the pole while lifting the body off the ground. Flex the hips, abduct the thighs, and fully extend the knees. Keep the pole between the thighs and facing the pubic bone to maintain a centralized body position while climbing up the pole hand over hand. Repeat.

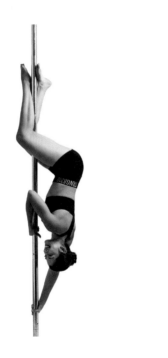

CATERPILLAR CLIMB

Begin with an inverted leg hold and grasp the pole with a two-handed strong hold grip. Maintain adducted legs. Support the chest on the pole, flex the knees to hip level, push the body away, and extend both elbows by shifting to a two-handed half grip. Bring the bottom toward the heels. Extend the knees to slide the legs on the pole. Repeat.

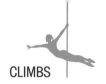

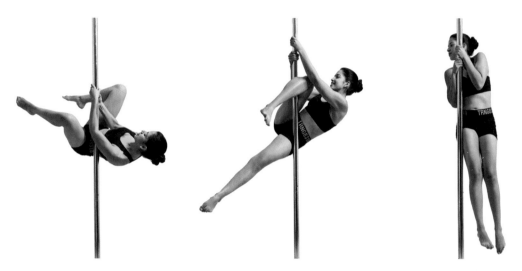

CONTINUOUS KNEE HOOK CLIMB

Begin with a body inversion. Hook the pole behind the far knee and hold the pole above the hooked knee. Release the leg hook and extend both knees, maintaining adducted legs parallel to pole. Engage the abdominal muscles to perform an aerial inversion and repeat.

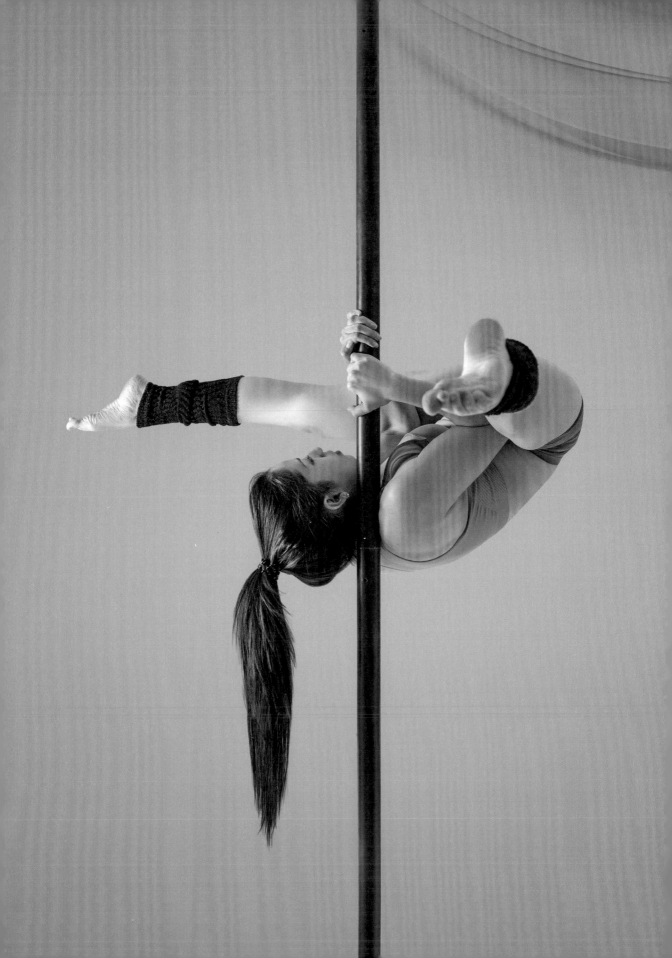

CHAPTER 7
SHOULDER MOUNTS

CHAPTER 7
SHOULDER MOUNTS

Shoulder mount inversions are transitional movements and tricks that require a great amount of core and arm strength. Shoulder mounts rely on hand and shoulder strength in order to reach a full-body inversion and execute the final stunt. Although much of the support comes from the upper fibers of the trapezius muscles, abdominal strength is also important as it allows inversions to take place while the legs assume different positions on or around the pole. This pole dance and fitness guide provides challengers with conditioning exercises in preparation for the execution of shoulder mount transitions, and it is necessary to consider the specific guidelines for improved technical comprehension. Basic inversions must be achieved prior to attempting shoulder mount stunts; abdominal and back muscles must develop in order to invert the body safely, maintain an aerial inverted straddle position, and avoid back arches that may increase injury risks. Performing jumps to engage a shoulder mount is counterproductive; these exercises must be gradually incorporated into conditioning and habitual training.

SHOULDER MOUNTS

- Beginner shoulder mount
- Hangman
- Shoulder mount tuck
- Scissor kick
- Shoulder mount attitude
- Shoulder mount straddle
- Shoulder mount pencil
- Shoulder dismount horizontal plank

- Shoulder mount plank passé hold
- Shoulder mount jack knife
- Shoulder mount lock
- Shoulder mount split through
- Princess grip straddle
- Aerial shoulder mount
- Shoulder mount bounce descent
- Shoulder mount pop

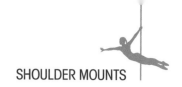

SHOULDER MOUNTS

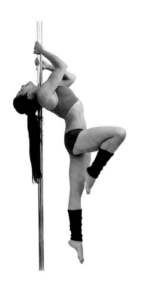

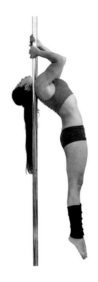

BEGINNER SHOULDER MOUNT

Comfortably support the shoulder (trapezius) on the pole, ensuring a two-handed cup grip. Contract abdominal muscles, flexing either knee toward the chest. Suspend the body on the pole and hold this position. The opposite knee remains extended and supported on the ground, if necessary.

HANGMAN

Comfortably support the shoulder (trapezius) on the pole, ensuring a two-handed cup grip. Maintain shoulder support and contract the abdominal muscles, suspending the body on pole. Both knees remain fully extended and the legs remain adducted. Hold this position.

SHOULDER MOUNT TUCK

Comfortably support the shoulder (trapezius) on the pole, ensuring a two-handed cup grip. Flex the knees, maintaining leg adduction. Contract the abdominal muscles to bring the flexed knees to the chest and hold this position.

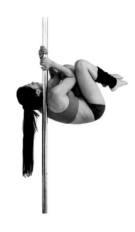

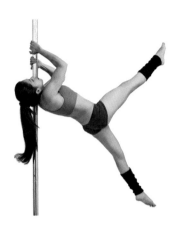

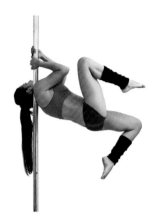

SCISSOR KICK

Comfortably support the shoulder (trapezius) on the pole, ensuring a two-handed cup grip. Contract the abdominal muscles and swing one leg up, performing a slight jump. The opposite leg follows. Both knees remain fully extended. Return to the starting position and repeat.

SHOULDER MOUNT ATTITUDE

Comfortably support the shoulder (trapezius) on the pole, ensuring a two-handed cup grip. Flex the knees, maintaining leg adduction. Contract the abdominal muscles to bring the flexed knees to the chest. One thigh should be flexed at the hip to 90 degrees, while the opposite knee flexes back at the thigh. Hold this position.

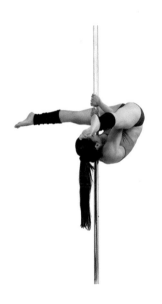

SHOULDER MOUNT STRADDLE

Comfortably support the shoulder (trapezius) on the pole, ensuring a two-handed cup grip. Maintain extended and abducted legs and contract the abdominal muscles to bring the legs toward the chest, and then extend them past the head. Hold this position.

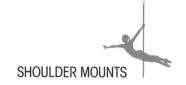

SHOULDER MOUNT PENCIL

Comfortably support the shoulder (trapezius) on the pole, ensuring a two-handed cup grip. Maintain adducted legs and contract the abdominal muscles to bring the flexed knees to the chest. Hold this position. When confident, extend both knees, keeping the legs adducted parallel to the pole. Maintain proper body alignment.

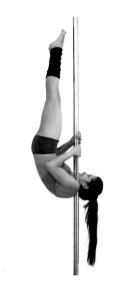

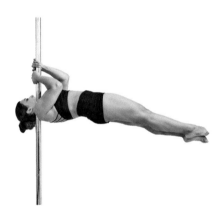

SHOULDER DISMOUNT HORIZONTAL PLANK

Comfortably support the shoulder (trapezius) on the pole, ensuring a two-handed cup grip. Maintain adducted legs and contract the abdominal muscles to bring the flexed knees to the chest. Hold this position. Extend both knees, keeping the legs adducted parallel to the pole. When confident, gradually lower the trunk and legs toward the horizontal plane while maintaining proper body alignment.

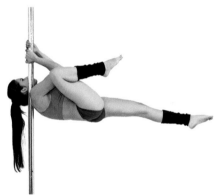

SHOULDER MOUNT PLANK PASSÉ HOLD

Comfortably support the shoulder (trapezius) on the pole, ensuring a two-handed cup grip. Maintain adducted legs and contract the abdominal muscles to bring the flexed knees to the chest. Hold this position. Extend both knees, keeping the legs adducted parallel to the pole. When confident, flex one knee toward the chest while the opposite knee remains fully extended to gradually lower the trunk toward the horizontal plane while maintaining proper body alignment and leg position.

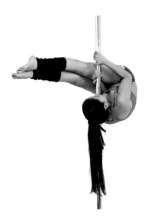

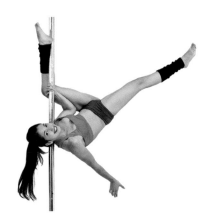

SHOULDER MOUNT JACK KNIFE

Comfortably support the shoulder (trapezius) on the pole, ensuring a two-handed cup grip. Maintain adducted thighs and contract the abdominal muscles to bring the flexed knees to the chest. Extend both knees, keeping the legs adducted parallel to the pole. When confident, turn the hips sideways and extend the legs lateral to pole. Hold this position.

SHOULDER MOUNT LOCK

Comfortably support the shoulder (trapezius) on the pole, ensuring a two-handed cup grip. Maintain adducted thighs and contract the abdominal muscles to bring the flexed knees to the chest. Extend both knees, keeping the legs adducted and parallel to the pole. When confident, support the near ankle and calf on the pole. Lower the hips and fully extend the far leg. Release the far hand grip and hold this position.

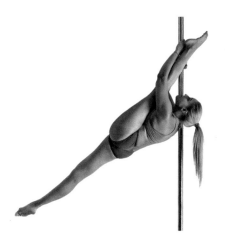

SHOULDER MOUNT SPLIT THROUGH

Assume a shoulder mount tuck position, ensuring a two-handed cup grip. When confident, place the far knee between the arms and support the ankle on the pole. Fully extend both knees and lower the hips, assuming a split position.

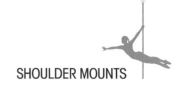

PRINCESS GRIP STRADDLE

Comfortably support the shoulder (trapezius) on the pole, ensuring a two-handed princess grip. Keep the legs abducted wider than the hips and contract the abdominal muscles to bring the pelvis to the pole. Hold this position.

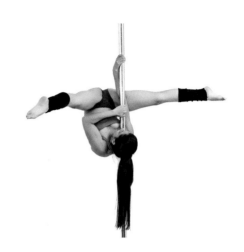

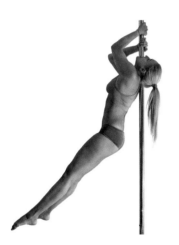

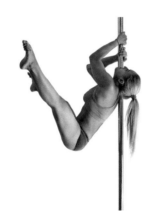

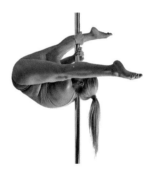

AERIAL SHOULDER MOUNT

From a back supported aerial stunt, support the shoulder (trapezius) on the pole, ensuring a two-handed cup grip. The legs should be adducted to secure grip on the pole. When confident, contract the abdominal muscles to rapidly suspend the body and raise the hips to bring the pelvis toward the pole. Hold this position.

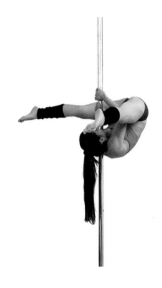

SHOULDER MOUNT BOUNCE DESCENT

Comfortably support the shoulder (trapezius) on the pole, ensuring a two-handed cup grip. Keep the legs extended and abducted while contracting the abdominal muscles to bring the legs toward the chest and fully extend the knees. When confident, spring the hips up to descend, using a hand-over-hand climbing motion. Continuously repeat the exercise. Return to the starting position and practice on the opposite side.

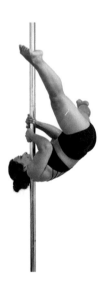

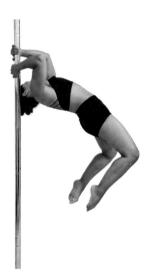

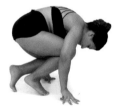

SHOULDER MOUNT POP

Comfortably support the shoulder (trapezius) on the pole, ensuring a two-handed cup grip. Keep the legs extended and abducted while contracting the abdominal muscles to bring the legs toward the chest and fully extend the knees. When confident, strongly spring the hips and legs up to jump toward the ground. Land safely with feet plantar flexed.

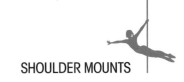

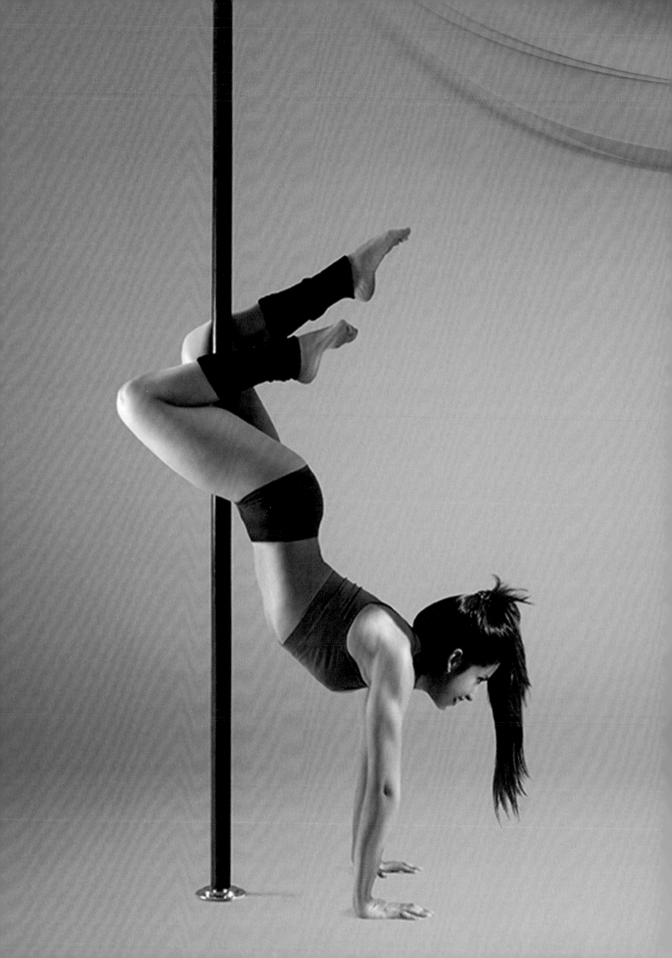

CHAPTER 8
HANDSTANDS

CHAPTER 8
HANDSTANDS

Handstands and forearm-supported stands are essential parts of pole dance performance (as well as being considered acrobatic tricks), serving as a transition from one movement to another and embellishing choreography and pole dance routines. Handstands may also be performed as conditioning exercises. Placing body support on the hands from a vertical inverted position, handstands force challengers to maintain stability and balance by engaging significant muscle groups, such as the pectorals, shoulders, back, glutes, legs, and abdominals. Handstand practice not only contributes to challengers' performances by strengthening muscles and improving skill development, it also positively influences metabolism and stimulates the endocrine system, pituitary gland, and thyroid glands. By maintaining an inverted position of the body, gravity increases blood flow and oxygen to the head, providing beneficial effects to the performer's progress, as well as to their physical, emotional, and mental condition.

Proper body alignment, balance, and shoulder, arm, wrist, and abdominal muscle strength will develop progressively through continuous conditioning and postural training. This pole dance and fitness guide offers challengers a selection of handstands and forearm-supported stands to be performed gradually, moving from basic to more challenging positions. It is highly recommended to incorporate handstand exercises to regular training sessions, keeping in mind technical guidelines in order to achieve a safer and more effective practice.

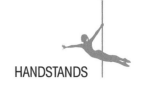

HANDSTANDS

- Forearm support pencil
- Forearm support fang
- Forearm support attitude
- Forearm support bow and arrow
- Forearm support passé
- Pole handstand

- Butterfly handstand
- Bridged handstand
- Floor handspring
- One-handed handstand
- Handstand split
- Tucked handstand

HANDSTANDS

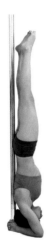

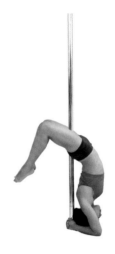

FOREARM SUPPORT PENCIL

Kneel facing the pole and use a cup grip at the base of the pole, supporting the forearms on the ground with elbows pointed out for stability. Bend the head forward between the forearms and extend the legs, raising the hips to walk the toes toward the pole. Once the back is fully supported on the pole, swing one leg up followed by the other.

FOREARM SUPPORT FANG

Kneel facing the pole and use a cup grip at the base of the pole, supporting the forearms on the ground with elbows pointed out for stability. Bend the head forward between the forearms, and extend legs, raising the hips to walk the toes toward the pole. Once the back is fully supported on the pole, lower the legs backwards while gradually arching the back and keeping the pole between the thighs.

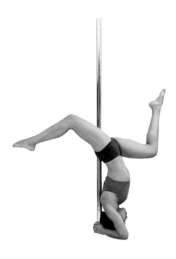

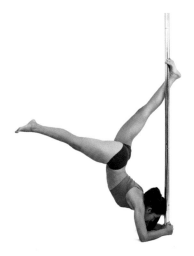

FOREARM SUPPORT ATTITUDE

Kneel facing the pole and use a cup grip at the base of the pole, supporting the forearms on the ground with elbows pointed out for stability. Bend the head forward between the forearms and extend the legs, raising the hips to walk the toes toward the pole. Once the back is fully supported on the pole, bend one leg forward and the opposite one backward with the knees flexed to 90 degrees.

FOREARM SUPPORT BOW AND ARROW

Kneel facing the pole and use a cup grip at the base of the pole, supporting the forearms on the ground with elbows pointed out for stability. Bend the head forward between the forearms and extend the legs, raising the hips to walk the toes toward the pole. Once the back is fully supported on the pole, maintain ankle flexion to secure the grip while moving the hips away from the pole. Opposite leg flexes forward in a straight position.

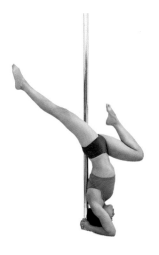

FOREARM SUPPORT PASSÉ

Kneel facing the pole and use a cup grip at the base of the pole, supporting the forearms on the ground with elbows pointed out for stability. Bend the head forward between the forearms and extend the legs, raising the hips to walk the toes toward the pole. Once the back is fully supported on the pole, flex one knee toward the chest while the opposite leg extends backward.

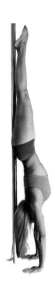

POLE HANDSTAND

Face the pole. Lean forward to support the palms on the ground, maintaining shoulder stability and alignment with the wrists and extended elbows. Raise the hips to walk the toes toward the pole. Swing the legs up, maintaining adduction and contact with the pole.

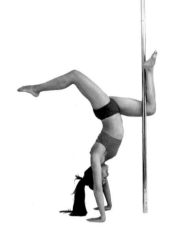

BUTTERFLY HANDSTAND

Begin the exercise in an inverted crucifix position. Gradually slide both legs down the pole to support the hands on the ground. The elbows remain fully extended and the chest is supported on the pole. Keep the legs adducted. When confident, separate the hips from the pole and flex the knees to hip level while supporting the calf on the pole and extending the opposite thigh back with knee flexion. Hold this position.

BRIDGED HANDSTAND

Assume a layback position with crossed ankles. Holding the pole in a two-handed iguana grip, carefully slide down the pole while maintaining grip with the legs. Make sure the glutes are positioned below hand level and elbows are extended. Extend the arms overhead while sliding the body down to support the palms on the ground. When confident, flex the upper knee and support the ankle on the opposite thigh. The opposite leg remains fully extended. Hold this position.

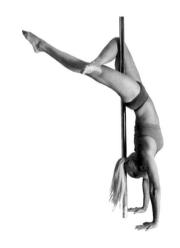

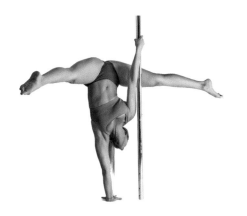

FLOOR HANDSPRING

Assume a position facing sideways to the pole. Bend forward to place the far hand on the ground. With the opposite hand, grasp the pole using a one-hand iguana grip with the shoulder internally rotated. Swing the legs up while contracting abdominal muscles to maintain leg adduction parallel to the pole. When confident, abduct the extended legs assume a middle split position.

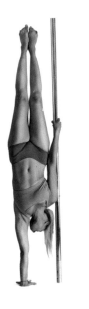

ONE-HANDED HANDSTAND

Assume a position facing sideways to the pole. Bend forward to place the far hand on the ground. With the opposite hand, grasp the pole using a one-hand iguana grip with the shoulder internally rotated. When confident, swing the legs up while contracting the abdominal muscles to maintain leg adduction parallel to the pole.

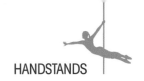

HANDSTAND SPLIT

Assume a position facing sideways to the pole. Bend forward to place the far hand on the ground. With the opposite hand, grasp the pole using a one-hand iguana grip with the shoulder internally rotated. Swing the legs up while contracting the abdominal muscles to maintain leg adduction parallel to the pole. When confident, take one leg forward and the opposite leg backward. Maintain body balance and legs in the horizontal plane.

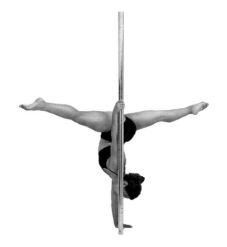

TUCKED HANDSTAND

Assume a position facing sideways to the pole. Bend forward to place the far hand on the ground. With the opposite hand, grasp the pole using a one-hand iguana grip with the shoulder internally rotated. Swing the legs up while contracting the abdominal muscles to maintain leg adduction parallel to the pole. When confident, bend the knees toward the chest and hold this position.

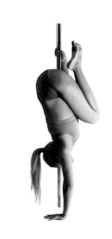

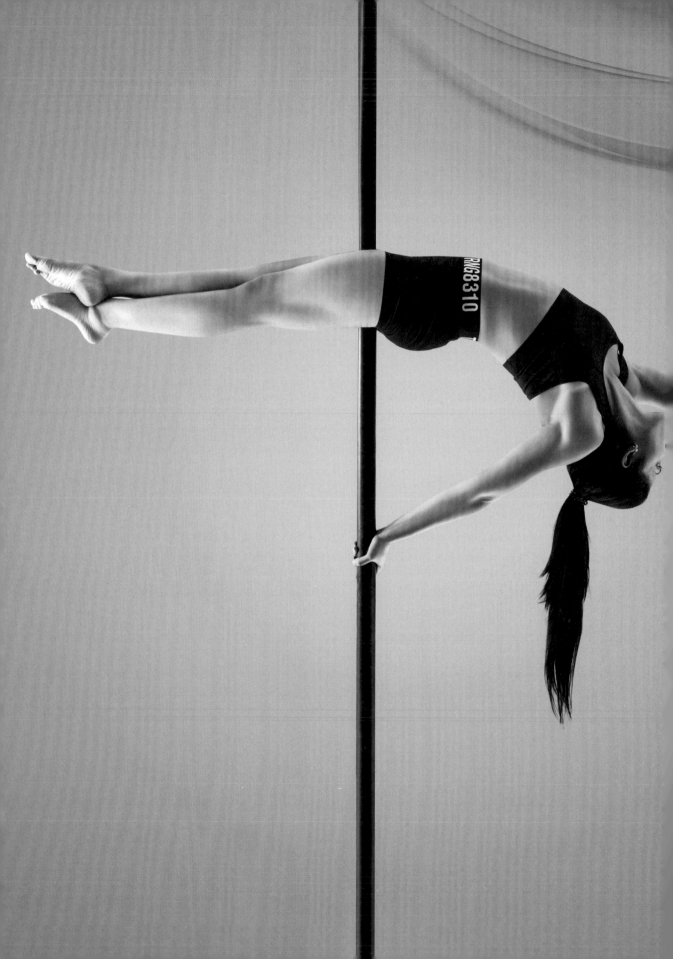

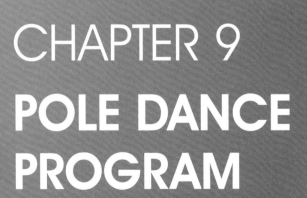

CHAPTER 9
POLE DANCE
PROGRAM

CHAPTER 9
POLE DANCE PROGRAM

This program includes three levels of performance: basic, intermediate, and advanced. Each level illustrates a variety of tricks, figures, and movements with descriptive technical notes for practical use and better understanding.

The moves described in this program are to be performed progressively as each trick, figure, and movement prepare the challenger for the next in the sequence. The terminology for each trick and figure is based on rigorous research in pole dance studios around the world and represents the technical and commonly used names related to the qualities of the movements and poses. Challengers should consult other sources of information because certain tricks might be recognized by different names, allowing an increased comprehension. However, in order to avoid confusion, it is recommended to select a single term to be associated with each trick.

Reviewing the chapter on positions and pole principles, as well as the pole commandments and sins, is mandatory before each session, and be sure to dedicate time for warm-up, stretching, and workout exercises for a safer and improved performance. Likewise, the amount of time spent at each level will depend on each person's development and the type, intensity, and frequency of the training.

It's also important to practice the tricks on both sides of your body; it's common that one side of your body might be more developed than the other, making tricks easier to perform on that side and harder on the opposite one; however, the goal is to increasingly reinforce skill training on both sides to be equally capable of performing the tricks. Regarding the pole type to be used, it is recommended that you train using both the static and the spinning poles.

Attendance at a professional dance studio is also highly recommended as well as the presence of a certified pole dance instructor at all times.

BASIC

The basic level is the primary introduction to the learning and instructive process. It introduces performers to the basic movements, stunts, and spins performed on the pole, and guides them to make their first approach to the fitness program. It allows challengers to assimilate new physical demands that will progressively develop strength and the comprehensive development of technical aspects and skills, and to encounter their movement awareness and sensibility, acquiring and increasing self-confidence as well as the desired movement fluency and accuracy.

An index of stunts and spins is provided to facilitate the reader's training and preparation. The basic level includes beginner spins that may be complemented by transitional movements in order to create combinations and transitions from one to the other. Be sure to consider the importance of an optimistic approach to every practice; the process is continuous and progressive, and results are a certainty.

BASIC PROGRAM

- Pole walk
- Step around
- Bridge
- Spider spin
- Swan slide
- Fireman spin
- One-hand lateral slide
- Fireman knee and ankle hold
- Windmill spin
- Fireman knee hold
- Fireman spin pike
- Half-pike spin
- Attitude spin
- Fireman kick
- Hook
- Half front hook
- Front hook
- Knee hook spin
- Back hook
- Side hold (hand off)
- Side hold
- Spinning chair
- Pike chair
- Forward attitude
- Pedaling chair
- Backward attitude

- Tinkerbell
- Hollywood spin
- Juliette spin
- Carousel spin
- Dolphin
- Boomerang straddle spin
- Tucked cradle spin
- Half cradle spin
- Straddle cradle spin
- Stand on pole
- Back support tuck
- Back support concorde
- Reverse grab attitude
- Reverse grab fang
- Reverse grab pencil
- Post spin
- Reverse grab spin straddle
- Apprentice
- Corkscrew
- Pencil spin forearm grip
- Ballerina
- Aerial leg hold (crucifix)
- Pendulum
- Reverse grab spin
- Thigh hold
- Forward fold

- Seated tuck
- Pike pole sit
- Seated side tuck
- Pike sit (elbow grip)
- Crossed pole sit
- Frontal pole sit
- Hip lock tuck/drama queen
- Hip lock pike
- Peter Pan
- Plank (hand on top)
- Snake
- Wrist sit
- Scissors
- Sultress
- Daphne
- Daphne variation
- Layback plank (lower support)
- Lean back stand
- Frog
- Harp
- Soldier
- Genevieve
- Front armpit hold attitude (hood ornament)
- Skater

- Pole hug (embrace)
- Cradle split
- Pole hug fang (embrace)
- Pencil spin baseball grip
- Pole hug (one-arm embrace)
- Scissor spin baseball grip
- Super girl
- Rocket man
- Yogini
- Twisted yogini
- Armpit hold straddle (teddy)
- Armpit hold (teddy variation)
- Layback (crossed knee)
- Basic rainbow
- Closed crossed knee release
- Stargazer
- Liberty
- Shishi spin
- Layback crossed ankle
- Pixie
- Crescent moon
- Bow and arrow
- Inverted pencil
- Iguana fang

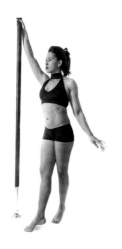

POLE WALK

Points of support: Hands

Main focus: Maintain feet plantar flexed throughout the exercise along with an upright posture and shoulder stability while walking around the pole with either grip. Flex the knees toward the back or slide the toes with every step. To change course, the far leg comes near the pole and the body rotates while simultaneously changing the hand grip.

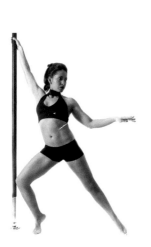
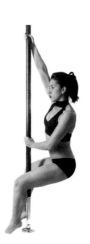
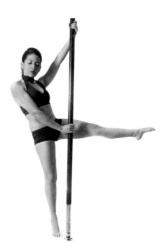

STEP AROUND

Points of support: Hands

Main focus: Start with a pole walk and maintain feet plantar flexed throughout the exercise. Keep an upright posture and maintain shoulder stability. Hold the pole with a split grip and rotate the far leg forward in a clockwise motion on the ground until it reaches the opposite foot. Push away from the pole with a lower hand grip.

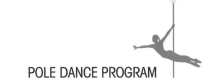

BRIDGE

Points of support: Hand and flank

Main focus: Maintain feet plantar flexed throughout the exercise. Grasp the pole with a one-hand strong hold and lean back, gradually extending the arm. Back flexibility is required. When confident, release the far hand's grip and reach for the floor, maintaining an arched back.

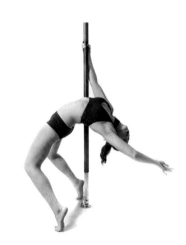

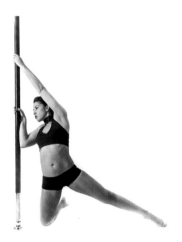
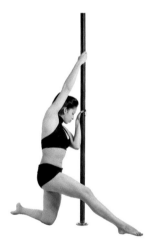
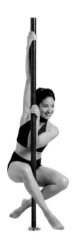

SPIDER SPIN

Points of support: Hands and forearm

Main focus: Maintain shoulder stability and forearm support. Rotate the far leg forward in a clockwise motion on the ground and flex the knees to hip level, crossing the legs for the duration of the spin.

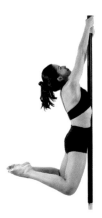

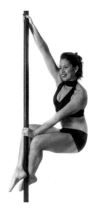

SWAN SLIDE

Points of support: Hands and abdomen

Main focus: Maintain a baseball grip on the pole. Fully contract the hamstrings and glutes. Both hips extend backwards, slightly wider than hip-width apart, and knees are flexed. Toes are in contact with each other.

FIREMAN SPIN

Points of support: Hands, anterior and posterior ankle

Main focus: With an upright posture and shoulder stability, maintain a split grip. With the pole between the knees, extend legs and keep ankles together. When confident, release the lower hand. Momentum technique is highly recommended.

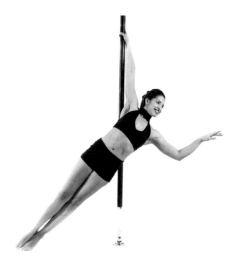

ONE-HAND LATERAL SLIDE

Points of support: Hand and feet

Main focus: Toes should be flexed throughout the whole exercise. Posture should be upright and shoulders stable. Grasp the pole with a basic grip and tilt the body to the front and then to the side of the pole. Gradually release the hand's grip, simultaneously sliding the inner foot's dorsum until it reaches the ground. Maintain body alignment throughout the exercise.

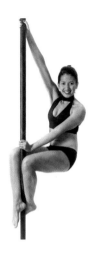

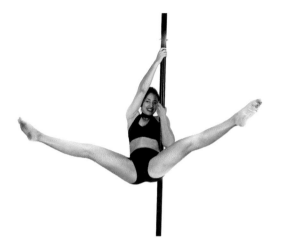

FIREMAN KNEE AND ANKLE HOLD

Points of support: hands, anterior and posterior ankle support.

Main focus: Upright posture and shoulders stability. Maintain a split grip. Strongly press knees and ankles to the pole. When confident, release lower hand. Momentum technique is highly recommended.

WINDMILL SPIN

Points of support: Hands, upper arm, and flank

Main focus: Maintain shoulder stability and a strong hold grip. Flex the hips with extended knees and abducted thighs. Apply hip support while the legs are apart in a clockwise rotation.

FIREMAN KNEE HOLD

Points of support: Hands, anterior and posterior ankle

Main focus: Maintain an upright posture and shoulder stability. Hold the pole with a split grip or a baseball grip. Strongly press the knees and ankles to the pole. When confident, release the ankle support and lift the feet toward the buttocks. Momentum technique is highly recommended. Ankles are in contact with each other.

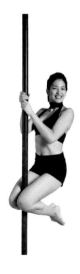

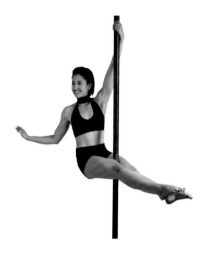

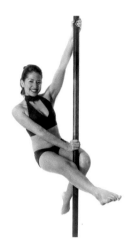

FIREMAN SPIN PIKE

Points of support: Hand and thighs

Main focus: Maintain shoulder stability and a split grip on the pole. Legs are extended at hip level with the thighs adducted and strongly pressed to the pole. When confident, release the lower hand. Ankles are in contact with each other.

HALF-PIKE SPIN

Points of support: Hands, thighs, and knees

Main focus: Maintain shoulder stability and a split grip on the pole. Legs are extended at hip level with the thighs adducted and knees strongly pressed to the pole. When confident, extend the far leg and lift the opposite foot toward the buttocks. When confident, release lower hand.

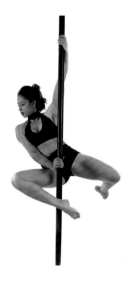

ATTITUDE SPIN

Points of support: Hands

Main focus: Maintain shoulder stability and preserve a two-handed half grip. Legs are abducted with one internally rotated and the other externally rotated. The pole is between the thighs facing the pubic bone. Momentum technique is highly recommended.

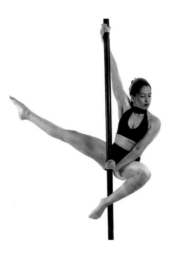

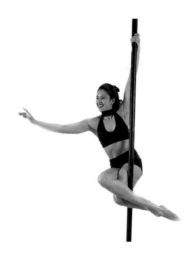

FIREMAN KICK

Points of support: Hands and posterior ankle

Main focus: Maintain an upright posture and shoulder stability. Maintain a split grip on the pole. The pole is between thighs facing pubic bone. Slightly bend the trunk laterally to the supporting leg. The opposite leg is abducted and kicks upward. Basic momentum technique is highly recommended.

HOOK

Points of support: Hands and back of knee hook

Main focus: Maintain shoulder stability and a back of knee hook with the near leg. Hips lean back to the pole and the outer leg crosses over. When confident, release the lower hand.

HALF FRONT HOOK

Points of support: Hands and back of knee hook

Main focus: Maintain an upright posture and shoulder stability. Ensure hip is in contact to the pole and grasp it using a two-handed half grip. The back of the knee of the near leg hooks on the pole. Adduct the near thigh and abduct the far leg sideways to the pole with the knee extended. When confident, release the lower hand.

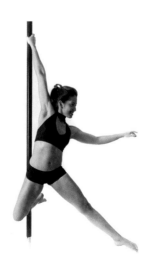

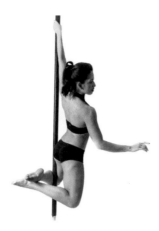

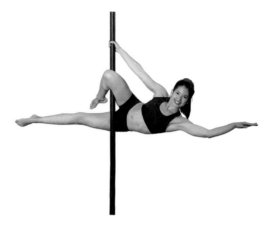

FRONT HOOK

Points of support: Hands and back of knee

Main focus: Maintain an upright posture and shoulder stability. Stand beside the pole with the hip in contact with it. Grasp the pole with a two-handed half grip. The back of the near leg's knee hooks around the pole with the hips positioned forward. Keep the knees apart and the ankles crossed. When confident, release the lower hand.

KNEE HOOK SPIN

Points of support: Hands and back of knee

Main focus: Extend the trunk in the horizontal plane. Hook the back of the near leg's knee around the pole. Grasp the pole with a two-handed full bracket split grip and support the back of the thigh on the pole. Lean the trunk forward to spin and lift the far leg off the floor. When confident, release the lower hand.

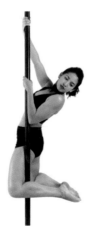

BACK HOOK

Points of support: Hands and back of knee

Main focus: Ensure an upright posture and shoulder stability. Stand beside the pole, with the hips and near leg in contact with it. Hook the back of the near leg's knee around the pole. Maintain a strong hold grip with the knees flexed 90 degrees and the toes in contact with each other. When confident, release the lower hand.

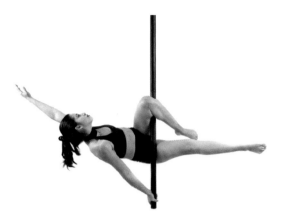 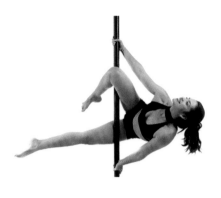

SIDE HOLD (HAND OFF)

Points of support: Hands and back of knee

Main focus: Extend the trunk in the horizontal plane. Hook the back of the near leg's knee around the pole. Grasp the pole with a two-handed full bracket split grip and support the back of the thigh on the pole. Lean the trunk forward to spin and lift the far leg off the floor. When confident, release the upper hand.

SIDE HOLD

Points of support: Hands and back of knee

Main focus: Hook the back of the near leg's knee around the pole above waist level and grasp the pole with a two-handed full bracket split grip. With the trunk extended in the horizontal plane, lift the far leg off the floor and press against the pole.

SPINNING CHAIR

Points of support: Hands

Main focus: Maintain an upright posture and shoulder stability. Grasp the pole with a split grip. Flex both knees at hip level. Basic momentum technique is highly recommended. Maintain a neutral pelvis.

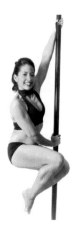

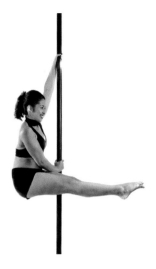

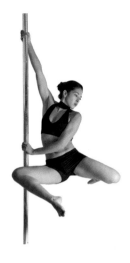

PIKE CHAIR

Points of support: Hands

Main focus: Maintain an upright posture and shoulder stability. Grasp the pole with a split grip. Flex both legs at hip level and adduct the thighs, extending both knees. Basic momentum technique is highly recommended. Maintain a neutral pelvis and keep the trunk positioned sideways to the pole.

FORWARD ATTITUDE

Points of support: Hands

Main focus: Maintain an upright posture and shoulder stability. Hold the pole with a two-handed half grip. Abduct the legs abducted with one internally rotated and the other externally rotated. Momentum technique is highly recommended.

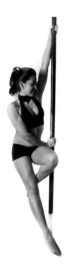

PEDALING CHAIR

Points of support: Hands.

Main focus: Maintain an upright posture and shoulder stability. Hold the pole with a split grip and flex both knees at hip level. Maintain a neutral pelvis and repetitively rotate the legs forward, pedaling in a steady, rhythmic pace. Basic momentum technique is highly recommended.

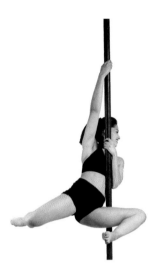

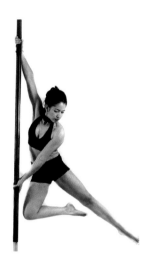

BACKWARD ATTITUDE

Points of support: Hands, chest, and thigh

Main focus: Maintain an upright posture and shoulder stability. Hold the pole with a two-handed strong hold grip. Abduct the legs abducted with one internally rotated and the other externally rotated. The near thigh, forearm, and chest are supported on the pole. Momentum technique is highly recommended.

TINKERBELL

Points of support: Hands

Main focus: Maintain an upright posture and shoulder stability. Position the body beside the pole and grasp it with a two-handed full bracket split grip. Maintain hip flexion and laterally rotate with the knee pointed out. The far leg extends sideways.

HOLLYWOOD SPIN

Points of support: Hands, posterior ankle, and calves

Main focus: Maintain shoulder stability and grasp the pole in a split grip. Initiate the spin by stabilizing the far ankle on the pole; flex the hips and extend the near knee. Repeat the movement counterclockwise. The pole is between the thighs, facing the pubic bone. Basic momentum technique is highly recommended.

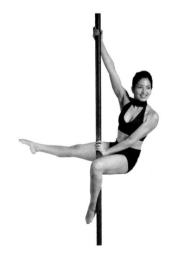

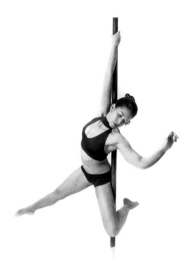

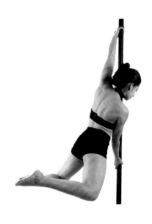

JULIETTE SPIN

Points of support: Hands and back of knee

Main focus: Maintain an upright posture and shoulder stability. Position the body beside the pole. Acquire momentum by extending the inner leg forward while drifting the pelvis away and hooking the back of the far leg's knee around the pole. Use a two-handed reverse grab followed by a one-hand twisted grip, and, when confident, release the lower hand.

CAROUSEL SPIN

Points of support: Hands

Main focus: Maintain shoulder stability. Grasp the pole with a two-handed full bracket split grip. Both hips extend backward. The knees are parted and flexed 90 degrees. Toes are in contact with each other.

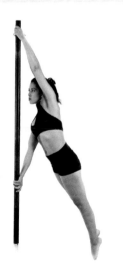

DOLPHIN

Points of support: Hands

Main focus: Hold the pole with a two-handed full bracket split grip. Both hips extend backward. The knees are adducted and extended. Keep the body pushed away from the pole. Toes are in contact with each other.

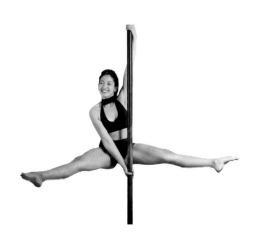

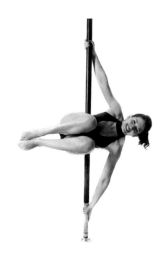

BOOMERANG STRADDLE SPIN

Points of support: Hands

Main focus: Ensure shoulder stability and hold the pole with a two-handed full bracket split grip. Flex the hips while keeping the thighs abducted and the knees fully extended. The pole should be between the thighs facing pubic bone. Maintain a centralized body position.

TUCKED CRADLE SPIN

Points of support: Hands, lower abdomen, and upper thighs

Main focus: Grasp the pole with a two-handed full bracket split grip, pressing the trunk and thighs against the pole. Bring the knees toward the chest, keeping the trunk in the horizontal plane.

HALF CRADLE SPIN

Points of support: Hands, lower abdomen, and upper thighs

Main focus: Grasp the pole with a two-handed full bracket split grip. Press the trunk and thighs against the pole. Bring the knees toward the chest, keeping the trunk in the horizontal plane. When confident, extend the lower knee.

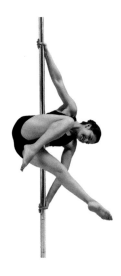

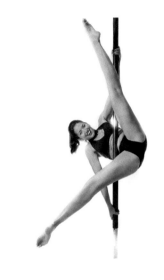

STRADDLE CRADLE SPIN

Points of support: Hands, lower abdomen, and upper thighs

Main focus: Grasp the pole using a two-handed full bracket split grip. Press the trunk and thighs against the pole. Bring the knees toward the chest, keeping the trunk in the horizontal plan. When confident, abduct the legs and fully extend the knees.

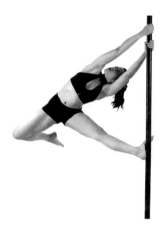

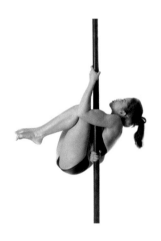

STAND ON POLE

Points of support: Hands and foot plantar

Main focus: Grasp the pole with a baseball grip. Place the sole of the foot on the pole with the knee extended. Rotate the body laterally, keeping the opposite leg abducted and the knee flexed backward.

BACK SUPPORT TUCK

Points of support: Hands, forearm, upper arm, and flank

Main focus: Maintain shoulder stability. Grasp the pole with a two-handed baseball back support grip. Support the back on the forearm and tuck the knees to chest level.

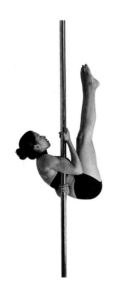

BACK SUPPORT CONCORDE

Points of support: Hands, forearm, upper arm, and flank

Main focus: Maintain shoulder stability and grasp the pole with a two-handed baseball back support grip. Support the back on the forearm and tuck the knees to chest level. When confident, extend both knees up.

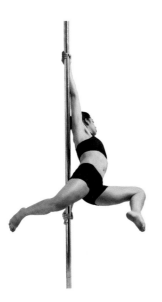

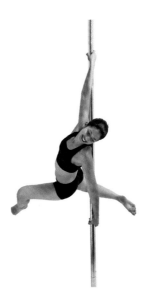

REVERSE GRAB ATTITUDE

Points of support: Hands

Main focus: Maintain an upright posture and shoulder stability and grasp the pole with a two-handed reverse grab grip. Abduct the legs with one internally rotated and the other externally rotated. Momentum technique is highly recommended.

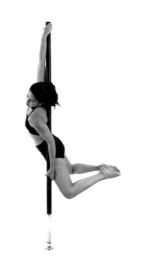

REVERSE GRAB FANG

Points of support: Hands, arms, and flank

Main focus: Maintain an upright posture and shoulder stability. Grasp the pole with a two-handed reverse grab grip. Both hips extend backward past the pole. The knees are apart and flexed 90 degrees. The hip is supported on pole and toes in contact with each other. Momentum technique is highly recommended.

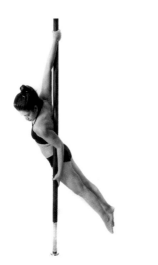

REVERSE GRAB PENCIL

Points of support: Hands, arms, and flank

Main focus: Maintain an upright posture and shoulder stability. Grasp the pole with a two-handed reverse grab grip. Both thighs extend back, and the hamstrings and glutes are fully contracted. Extend the knees backward past the pole and ankles in contact with each other. Momentum technique is highly recommended.

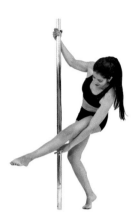
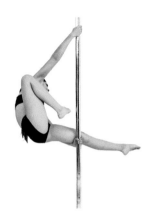
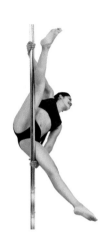

POST SPIN

Points of support: Hands, hamstrings, and back of knee

Main focus: Grasp the pole at knee level with a two-handed full bracket split grip and support the back of the far leg's knee on the wrist. Lean forward to spin and bring the near leg through (between the near arm and far leg). Both hamstrings are supported on the pole and the legs are fully extended.

REVERSE GRAB SPIN STRADDLE

Points of support: Hands

Main focus: Maintain an upright posture and shoulder stability. Grip the pole with a two-handed reverse grab grip. Both thighs extend back, and the hamstrings and glutes are fully contracted. Extend the legs backward and maintain a centralized body position. Momentum technique is highly recommended.

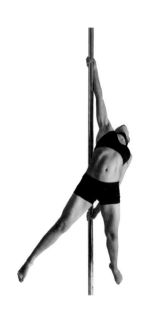

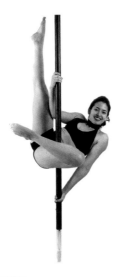

APPRENTICE

Points of support: Hands, abdomen, and thighs

Main focus: Grasp the pole with a two-handed full bracket split grip. Press the trunk and thighs against the pole. When confident, abduct and extend the upper leg parallel to the pole.

CORKSCREW

Points of support: Hands, upper arm, and flank

Main focus: Maintain shoulder stability and grasp the pole with a strong hold grip. Support the hips and flex the knees backward across the pole. Swing the legs forward to gain momentum and spin.

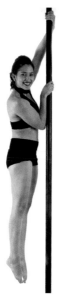

PENCIL SPIN FOREARM GRIP

Points of support: Hands and forearm

Main focus: Maintain an upright posture and shoulder stability. The basic climb is suggested. Grip the pole with the forearm, and fully contract the hamstrings and glutes. Both legs extend down parallel to the pole. Ankles are in contact with each other.

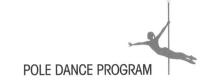

POLE DANCE PROGRAM

BALLERINA

Points of support: Hands, arms, flank, and thigh

Main focus: Maintain an upright posture and shoulder stability. Grasp the pole with a two-handed reverse grab grip. Both thighs extend back, and the hamstrings and glutes are fully contracted. Extend the knees backward past the pole and ankles in contact with each other. Wrap the near leg around the pole. Suggested spins are the single-handed chair, pendulum, or reverse grab spin. Momentum technique is highly recommended. When confident, release the lower hand grip.

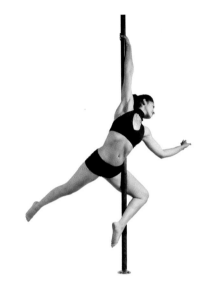

AERIAL LEG HOLD (CRUCIFIX)

Points of support: Hands, thighs, knees, anterior and posterior ankle

Main focus: Begin with a basic climb. Maintain an upright posture and shoulder stability. Fully contract the hamstrings and glutes. Press the knees and ankles strongly against the pole. The abdomen should be in contact with the pole. When confident, release both hands. Maintain a centralized body position.

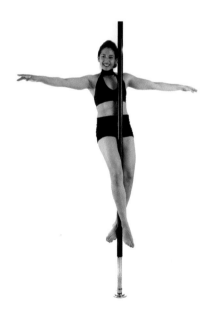

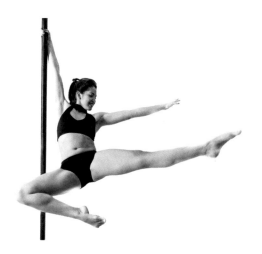

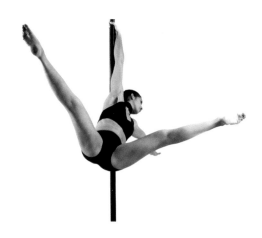

PENDULUM

Points of support: Hands

Main focus: Maintain an upright posture and shoulder stability. Acquire momentum by extending the far leg sideways while drifting the pelvis away. The near knee remains flexed while performing the body swing. Support the far hand to push the body away from the pole. When confident, extend the far arm.

REVERSE GRAB SPIN

Points of support: Hands

Main focus: Maintain an upright posture and shoulder stability. Swing the body, engaging the core muscles and extending both legs forward while drifting the pelvis away from the pole. Support the far hand to push the body away from the pole. When confident, extend the far arm.

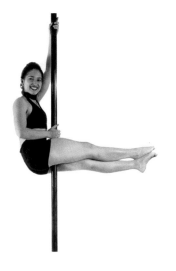

THIGH HOLD

Points of support: Hands and adductors

Main focus: Begin with a basic climb. With the knees flexed at the hip, the thighs adducted, and the legs fully extended forward, strongly press the thighs to the pole and cross the ankles. Maintain a centralized body position.

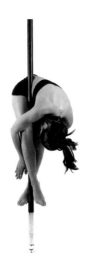

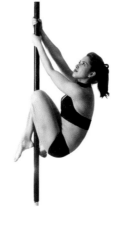

FORWARD FOLD

Points of support: Hands, thighs, knees, flank, anterior and posterior ankle

Main focus: Begin with a basic climb. Maintain an upright posture and shoulder stability. Fully contract the hamstrings and glutes, and strongly press the knees and ankles to the pole. The abdomen should be in contact with the pole. When confident, lean forward until the head reaches knee level.

SEATED TUCK

Points of support: Hands, knees, anterior and posterior ankle

Main focus: Begin with a basic climb. Fully contract the hamstrings and glutes, and strongly press the knees and ankles to the pole. Lean back to support the buttocks on the anterior calf. Maintain arm extension and a centralized body position.

PIKE POLE SIT

Points of support: Hands and thighs

Main focus: Begin with a basic climb. With the knees flexed at the hip and the thighs adducted and fully extended forward, strongly press the thighs to the pole and cross the ankles. Maintain a centralized body position. When confident, release either hand.

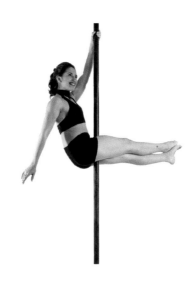

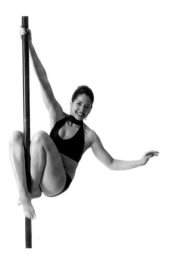

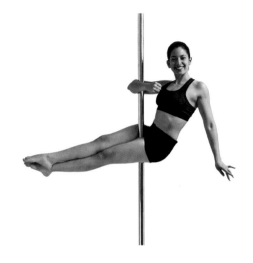

SEATED SIDE TUCK

Points of support: Hands, knees, anterior and posterior ankle

Main focus: Begin with a basic climb. Fully contract the hamstrings and glutes, and strongly press the knees and ankles to the pole. Lean back to support the buttocks on the anterior calf. Maintain arm extension and lean sideways. When confident, release either hand.

PIKE SIT (ELBOW GRIP)

Points of support: Hands and thighs

Main focus: Begin with a basic climb. With the knees flexed at the hip and the thighs adducted and fully extended forward, strongly press the thighs to the pole and cross the ankles. Maintain a centralized body position. When confident, stabilize one arm in an elbow grip and release the opposite hand.

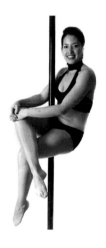

CROSSED POLE SIT

Points of support: Thighs

Main focus: Begin with a basic climb. The knees should be flexed at the hip, and the thighs adducted and strongly pressed to the pole. Cross the knees and lean slightly to one side to secure the thigh hold.

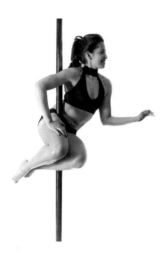

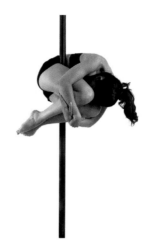

FRONTAL POLE SIT

Points of support: Thighs, flank, and underarm

Main focus: Begin with a basic climb. With the knees flexed at the hip and the thighs adducted and strongly pressed to the pole, lean the upper body slightly forward. When confident, lean forward past the pole so that it is anchored under the arm. The back of knees should be hooked strongly around the pole and flexed. Ankles are in contact with each other.

HIP LOCK TUCK/DRAMA QUEEN

Points of support: Thighs and flank

Main focus: Begin with a basic climb. The knees should be flexed at the hip, and the thighs adducted and strongly pressed to the pole. Lean the upper body to one side and tuck forward to knee level. Maintain this position, keeping the chest and trunk in contact with the thighs. Embrace the shins to secure the position.

HIP LOCK PIKE

Points of support: Thighs and flank

Main focus: Begin with a basic climb. Flex the knees at the hip, adduct the thighs, and press them strongly to the pole. Lean to one side and tuck forward to knee level. Maintain this position, keeping the chest and trunk in contact with the thighs. When confident, extend both knees and cross the ankles.

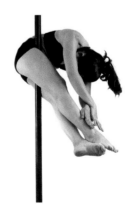

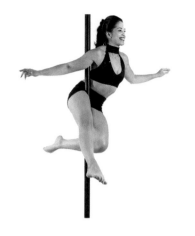

PETER PAN

Points of support: Thighs, flank, underarm, and back of knee

Main focus: The knees should be flexed at the hip, and the thighs adducted and strongly pressed to the pole. Lean forward and to one side, anchoring the under the near arm extended sideways. When confident, extend the inner leg and wrap the opposite one around the pole.

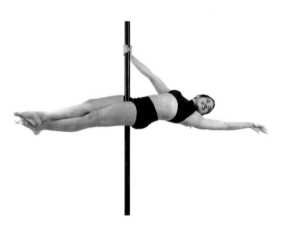

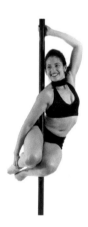

PLANK (HAND ON TOP)

Points of support: Hand and thighs

Main focus: Assume a cross ankle pole sit position. Lower the upper hand's grip, releasing the opposite hand, and lie back in the horizontal plane. Strongly adduct the thighs to the pole and keep the glutes contracted. Lower the ankles to secure the position.

SNAKE

Points of support: Hand, thighs, flank, and back of knee

Main focus: With the knees flexed at hip level, adduct the thighs and strongly press them to the pole. Lean forward and to one side. Wrap both legs around the pole and hold the ankle with the near arm. Reach the far arm overhead to the pole. Back flexibility and moderate contortion is required.

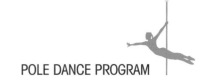

WRIST SIT

Points of support: Hands and forearm

Main focus: Begin with a basic climb and then assume a cross ankle pole sit position. Lower the upper hand's grip and use the opposite hand to hold the pole under the buttocks and in contact with the tailbone. When confident, flex both knees toward the chest and extend. Lean back, extending the arm. Maintain a centralized body position.

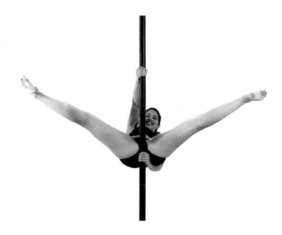

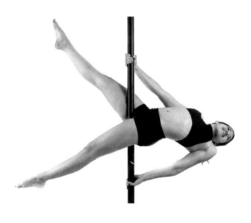

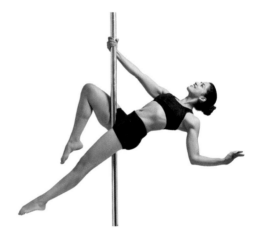

SCISSORS

Points of support: Hand and thighs

Main focus: Assume a cross ankle pole sit position. Lower the upper hand's grip, releasing the opposite hand, and lie back in the horizontal plane. Strongly adduct the thighs to the pole and keep the glutes contracted. Lower the ankles to secure the position. When confident, move the legs away from each other vertically. Maintain adducted thighs and moderate back arch.

SULTRESS

Points of support: Hand and thighs

Main focus: Assume a cross ankle pole sit position. Lower the upper hand's grip, releasing the opposite hand, and lie back in the horizontal plane. Strongly adduct the thighs to the pole and keep the glutes contracted. Lower the ankles to secure the position. When confident, flex either knee upward and extend the opposite leg downward.

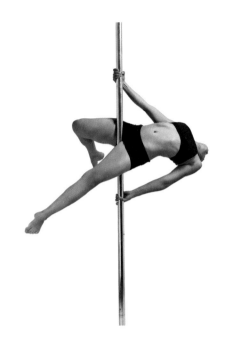

DAPHNE

Points of support: Hands and thighs

Main focus: Assume a cross ankle pole sit position. Lower the upper hand's grip and hold the pole under the glutes with opposite hand in a full bracket split grip, placing the arms equidistant from one another. Lie back to horizontal body alignment. Strongly press the thighs to the pole and keep the glutes contracted. When confident, turn the trunk sideways and flex the upper knee backward. The opposite leg remains fully extended.

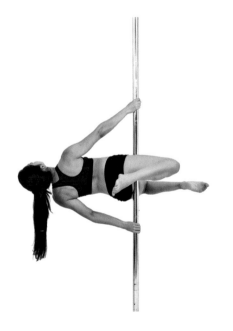

DAPHNE VARIATION

Points of support: Hands and thighs

Main focus: Assume a cross ankle pole sit position. Lower the upper hand's grip and hold the pole under the glutes with opposite hand in a full bracket split grip, placing the arms equidistant from one another. Lie back to horizontal body alignment. Strongly press the thighs to the pole and keep the glutes contracted. When confident, turn the trunk sideways and flex both knees; lower the thigh at the hip with the opposite knee flexed backward (both to 90 degrees).

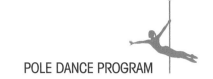

LAYBACK PLANK (LOWER SUPPORT)

Points of support: Hands and thighs

Main focus: Begin with a basic climb. Assume a cross ankle pole sit position. Lower the upper hand's grip and hold the pole under the glutes with the opposite hand in a full bracket split grip, placing the arms equidistant from one another. Lie back to the horizontal plane, slightly leaning sideways. Keep the glutes contracted and the thighs adducted. When confident, release the upper hand's grip. Secure this position by lowering the feet and the hand support while performing a moderate back arch.

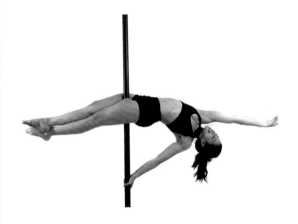

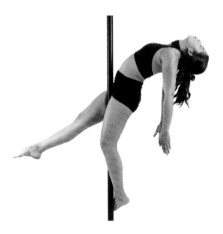

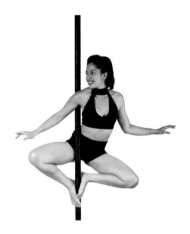

LEAN BACK STAND

Points of support: Hands, thighs, knees, anterior and posterior ankle

Main focus: Begin with a basic climb. Maintain an upright posture and shoulder stability. From a standing body position, raise the front leg to create a 30-degree angle with the pole. Keep the thighs adducted and gradually lean backward, releasing the grip with both hands.

FROG

Points of support: Feet's planter, flank, and underarm

Main focus: Begin with a Chinese climb. Lean the upper body forward and to the side to anchor the underarm on the pole, gradually sliding planters down the pole. Keep the thighs abducted and the knees flexed wider than the hips.

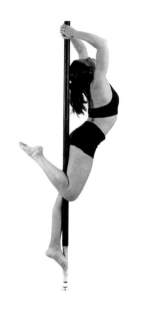

HARP

Points of support: Hamstrings, hips, armpit, back of knee, and foot dorsum

Main focus: Begin with an aerial leg hold or a side climb. Take a strong arm hold position, supporting the hip and the near leg hamstring on the pole. Strongly hook the back of the inner knee around the pole, maintaining the far foot's dorsum support. Anchor the pole under the near arm. When confident, take the body forward, supporting the tailbone on the pole. Maintain a two-handed double grip and bridge arch position.

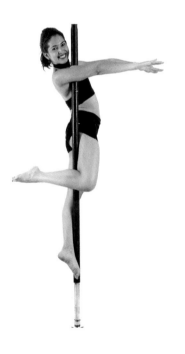

SOLDIER

Points of support: Hamstrings, hips, armpit, back of knee, and foot dorsum

Main focus: Begin with an aerial leg hold or side climb. Take strong arm hold position, supporting the inner hip and hamstring on the pole. Strongly hook the back of the inner knee around the pole, maintaining the far foot's dorsum support. Anchor the pole under the near arm. When confident, extend both arms forward.

GENEVIEVE

Points of support: Elbow, back of knee, hamstrings, hips, underarm, and foot dorsum

Main focus: Begin with a side climb. Strongly hook the back of the inner leg's knee on the pole. Support the inner leg's hamstring on the pole, and move the upper body to reach an elbow grip. When confident, reach the far leg out and hold it at knee level.

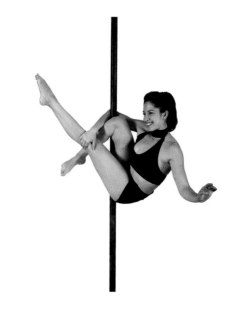

FRONT ARMPIT HOLD ATTITUDE (HOOD ORNAMENT)

Points of support: Hamstrings, hips, armpit, back of knee hook and foot dorsum

Main focus: Begin with an aerial leg hold or side climb. Take a strong hold arm position and support the inner hip and hamstring on pole. Strongly hook the back of the inner knee, maintain the far foot's dorsum support. The pole should be anchored under the near arm with the arms fully extended forward. When confident, lean back, extending the far arm backward.

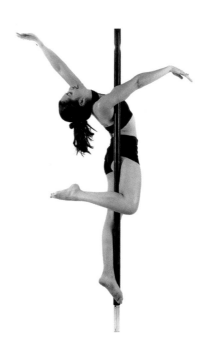

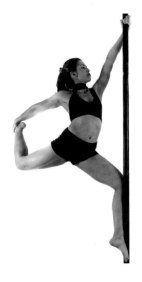

SKATER

Points of support: Hands, shin and posterior ankle

Main focus: Begin with an aerial leg hold. Slightly lower the hand grip, keeping the hamstrings and glutes fully contracted. Pull the body up, simultaneously moving the unsupported leg backward by holding the ankle. Maintain arm extension and a centralized body position.

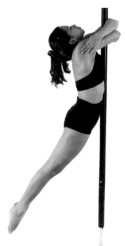

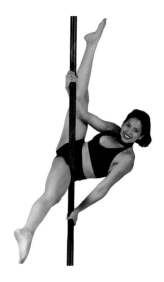

POLE HUG (EMBRACE)

Points of support: Elbows, chest, and abdomen

Main focus: Begin with an aerial leg hold. Maintain an upright posture and shoulder stability. Embrace the pole with both arms in an elbow grip and abduct the thighs backward wider than the hips. Keep the knees extended and maintain a centralized body position.

CRADLE SPLIT

Points of support: Hands, thighs, and groin

Main focus: Grasp the pole with a two-handed full bracket split grip. Press the trunk and thighs against the pole. When confident, abduct the thighs, maintaining near groin support on the pole. Rotate the near leg toward the pole in the horizontal plane while extending far leg up and out.

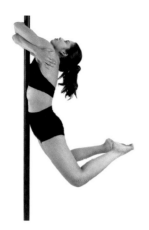

POLE HUG FANG (EMBRACE)

Points of support: Elbows, chest, and abdomen

Main focus: Begin with an aerial leg hold. Maintain an upright posture and shoulder stability. Embrace the pole with both arms in an elbow grip and abduct the thighs backward wider than the hips. Flex both knees and maintain a centralized body position.

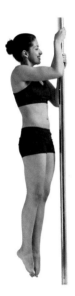

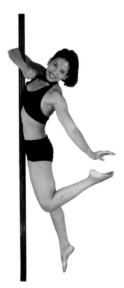

PENCIL SPIN BASEBALL GRIP

Points of support: Hands

Main focus: With an upright posture and shoulder stability, grasp the pole with a baseball grip. Fully contract the hamstrings and glutes and pull the body up. Hold the pose and preserve a centralized position with the body away from the pole. Ankles are in contact with each other.

POLE HUG (ONE-ARM EMBRACE)

Points of support: Elbows, chest, and abdomen

Main focus: Begin with an aerial leg hold. Maintain an upright posture and shoulder stability. Embrace the pole with both arms in an elbow grip and abduct the thighs backward wider than the hips. Extend or flex either knee. When confident, release one arm's elbow grip. Maintain a centralized body position.

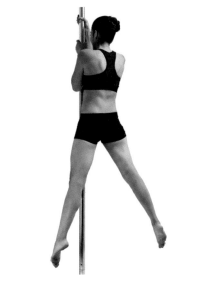

SCISSOR SPIN BASEBALL GRIP

Points of support: Hands

Main focus: With an upright posture and shoulder stability, grasp the pole with a baseball grip. Fully contract the hamstrings and glutes and pull the body up. Hold the pose and preserve a centralized position with the body away from the pole and the legs abducted.

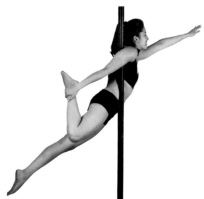

SUPER GIRL

Points of support: Underarm and flank

Main focus: Begin with an aerial leg hold position. Lean the trunk sideways and forward, anchoring the pole under the near arm. When confident, extend one leg backward and hold the ankle with the corresponding hand. It is highly recommended to keep the opposite hand's hold on the pole until confident enough to release grip.

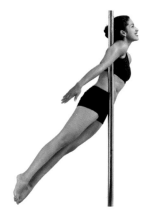

ROCKET MAN

Points of support: Underarm and flank

Main focus: Begin with an aerial leg hold position. Incline the upper body to one side and then forward, anchoring the pole under the near arm. When confident, extend both legs backward. Maintain an armpit hold with the trunk supported on the pole. It is recommended to keep the far hand's hold on the pole until confident to release grip.

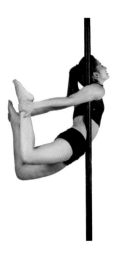

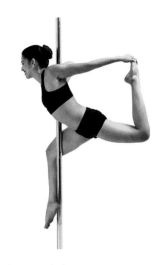

YOGINI

Points of support: Underarm and flank

Main focus: Begin with an aerial leg hold position. Incline the trunk sideways and forward, anchoring the pole under the near arm. When confident, extend both legs backward and hold each ankle with the corresponding hand. It is highly recommended to keep the far hand's hold on the pole or to begin the exercise with the Super Girl trick until confident to release grip.

TWISTED YOGINI

Points of support: Underarm, flank, and leg

Main focus: Begin with an aerial leg hold position. Move the upper trunk forward so that the pole is anchored under the near arm. When confident, raise the far leg backward and hold the ankle with the far hand, maintaining elbow extension.

ARMPIT HOLD STRADDLE (TEDDY)

Points of support: Hips, flank, and armpit

Main focus: Grasp the pole with an armpit grip and hip support. Abduct the inner hip with external rotation and hold it with the inner arm at knee level. When confident, extend the inner knee and raise the opposite leg, holding it with the ipsilateral hand at knee level. Keep both legs at hip level. Make sure the armpit hold is secure prior to abducting the legs.

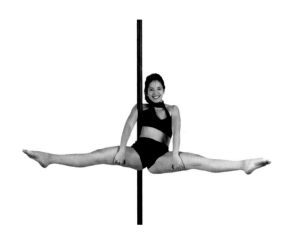

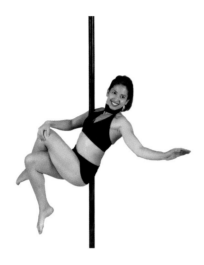

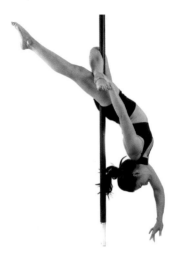

ARMPIT HOLD (TEDDY VARIATION)

Points of support: Hips, flank, and armpit

Main focus: Grasp the pole with an armpit grip and hip support. Flex both knees. Cross the far leg over the near thigh and hold it with the near hand at knee level. Make sure the armpit hold is secure prior to flexing the knees. When confident, release the far hand's grip.

LAYBACK (CROSSED KNEE)

Points of support: Thighs, back of knee, and tail bone

Main focus: Begin with a crossed ankle pole sit. With the upper knee flexed and supported on pole, hold the ankle with the opposite hand and lean back. Fully extend the opposite leg. When confident, release the hand's grip. Secure the position by maintaining contact between the extended leg and the flexed knee.

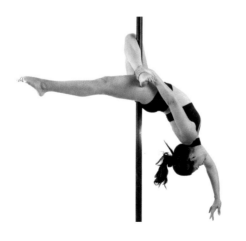

BASIC RAINBOW

Points of support: Thighs, back of knee, and tail bone

Main focus: Begin with a crossed ankle pole sit. With the upper knee flexed and supported on the pole, hold the ankle with the opposite hand and lean back. When confident, lower the extended leg to hip level.

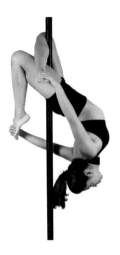

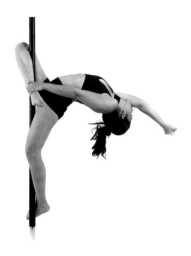

CLOSED CROSSED KNEE RELEASE

Points of support: Thighs, back of knee, and tail bone

Main focus: Begin with a crossed ankle pole sit. With the upper knee flexed and supported on the pole, hold the ankle with the opposite hand and lean back. When confident, reach to hold the opposite ankle. Secure the position by maintaining back arch.

STARGAZER

Points of support: Thighs and back of knee

Main focus: Begin with a layback crossed knee position. Slightly raise the upper trunk, while simultaneously sliding the lower leg down the pole until is fully extended. Secure the position by maintaining back arch and supporting the back of the knee on the pole.

LIBERTY

Points of support: Thighs, back of knee, and tail bone

Main focus: Begin with a crossed ankle pole sit. With the upper knee flexed and supported on the pole, hold the ankle with the opposite hand and lean backward. When confident, release the hand's grip and support it on the pole with a one hand down grip. Maintain proper body alignment.

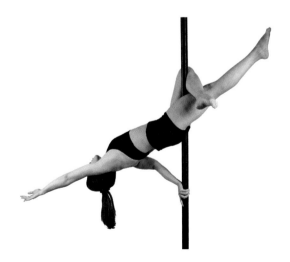

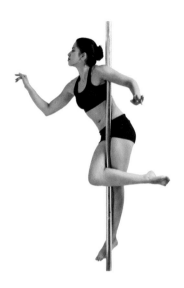 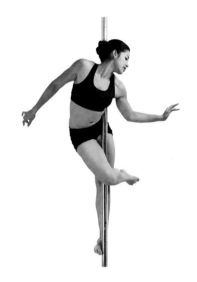

SHISHI SPIN

Points of support: Flank, upper back, thighs, shin, and foot dorsum

Main focus: Begin with an aerial leg hold position. Lean forward and flex the front knee to secure the position. Keep the back foot's dorsum supported on the pole.

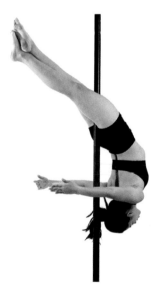

LAYBACK CROSSED ANKLE

Points of support: Thighs and tailbone

Main focus: Assume a cross-ankle pole sit position. Lower the upper hand's grip and hold the pole under the glutes with the opposite hand using a full bracket split grip and placing the arms equidistant from each other. Release the upper hand's grip and lean back to tailbone support. Release the lower hand support on pole and lean back. Keep the thighs adducted and the glutes contracted. When confident, extend both arms sideways.

PIXIE

Points of support: Foot dorsum, leg, and hands

Main focus: Assume a layback crossed ankle position. Keep the thighs adducted and the glutes contracted. Using a two-handed iguana grip, carefully slide the body down while maintaining a leg grip. The glutes should be positioned below hand level with the arms fully extended and the foot flexed to obtain a secure grip on the pole. When confident, flex the knee backward, keeping it in contact with the pole.

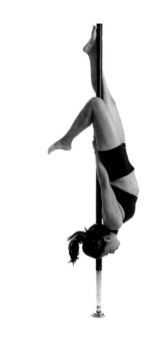

CRESCENT MOON

Points of support: Thighs, hands, and tailbone

Main focus: Assume a layback crossed ankle position. Keep the thighs adducted and the glutes contracted. When confident, perform a two-handed double bridge arch. Keep the legs in the horizontal plane by lowering the ankles. Back flexibility is required.

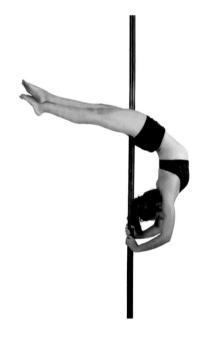

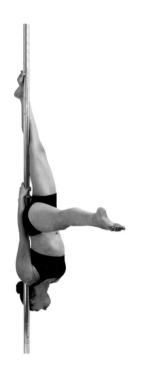

BOW AND ARROW

Points of support: Foot dorsum, leg, and hands

Main focus: Assume a layback crossed ankle position. Keep the thighs adducted and the glutes contracted. Using a two-handed iguana grip, carefully slide the body down, maintaining a leg grip. Position the glutes below hand level with the arms fully extended and the supported leg using a flexed ankle grip. When confident, move the opposite leg forward.

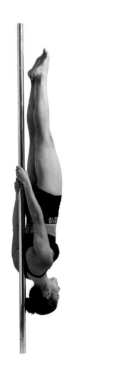

INVERTED PENCIL

Points of support: Foot dorsum, legs, and hands

Main focus: Assume a layback crossed ankle position. Keep the thighs adducted and the glutes contracted. Using a two-handed iguana grip, carefully slide the body down, maintaining a leg grip. Position the glutes below hand level with the arms fully extended and the upper leg's foot flexed and supported on the pole to ensure a safe grip. When confident, release the ankle grip and move the legs off the pole while maintaining body alignment.

IGUANA FANG

Points of support: Foot dorsum, leg, and hands

Main focus: Assume a layback crossed ankle position. Keep the thighs adducted and the glutes contracted. Using a two-handed iguana grip, carefully slide the body down, maintaining a leg grip. Position the glutes below hand level with the arms fully extended and the supported leg maintaining a flexed ankle grip. When confident, flex both knees backward, lean the head sideways, and support the trapezius on the pole. Maintain toes in contact with each other. Back flexibility is required.

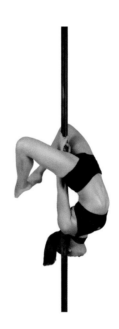

INTERMEDIATE

The intermediate level includes a selection of tricks and movement techniques as transitions from the basic to the advanced levels. Tricks and stunts will gradually increase their complexity; from grips to inverted body positions. It is necessary to fully perform all basic tricks to truly comprehend pole principles, body positions, and grips before advancing to the intermediate level. General workout routines must also be executed prior to the practice of intermediate pole dance stunts, in order to avoid risks of injuries, as well as suitable stretches to improve flexibility skills according to the specific tricks, movements and each challenger's level of performance. It is highly recommended to practice each of the stunts in isolation. Once the expected results are achieved, practice the movements and tricks combined within a routine. Post work out stretches are no less important, helping the body to cool down and relax muscles minimizing possible pain after the sessions, as well as developing flexibility skills to contribute to the process and a better execution of the stunts and movements.

INTERMEDIATE PROGRAM

- Inverted pencil V
- Cupid supported
- Dart
- Tuck drop
- Spaceflight
- Side V
- Inversion leg hold
- Inversion legs tucked
- Inverted crucifix
- Inversion legs extended
- Horizontal dismount
- Pencil full bracket split grip
- Air walk
- Basic inverted split
- Gemini attitude
- Top-handed outside knee hook
- Scorpion

- Scorpion attitude
- Scorpion hold (dragon)
- Scorpion flatliner
- Scorpion (foot hold)
- Static electric leg switch
- Cocoon
- Bow and arrow (one hand)
- Jasmine
- Dragonfly (Inverted thigh hold)
- Side pole straddle
- Dragonfly crossed
- Capezio
- Allegra
- Allegra split
- Doris spin
- Genie supported
- Doris split

- Cupid side
- Genie (no hands)
- Marley
- Marley flatliner
- Double knee hook release
- The Q
- Dangerous bird
- Hip hold passé
- Remi sit
- Inverted thigh hold tuck
- Remi sit (leg lock release)
- Lotus bridge (leg lock bridge)
- Inverted thigh hold pike
- Chinese pole sit
- Half jade
- Jumping straddle split
- Jade variation
- Jade
- Hercules (inverted hip hold straddle)
- Superman
- Superman crescent
- Superman scissors
- Superman (armpit grip)
- Seahorse
- Anastasia
- Titanic
- Thinker

- Star (flying ballerina)
- Vortex
- Superpain (no hands superman)
- Inverted D
- Butterfly split grip
- Handspring
- Butterfly twisted grip (legs extended)
- Split grip hang
- Twisted handspring
- Handspring straddle cup grip
- Twisted handspring pencil
- Chair (elbow grip)
- Handspring fang
- Pencil (elbow grip)
- Carousel spin (elbow grip)
- Cross grip tulip
- Tulip
- Alesia half split
- Crossbow (hands on pole)
- Cupid
- Teddy Buddha
- Brass monkey (inverted back hook)
- Brass monkey variation (inverted back hook)
- Eros
- Libellula variation
- Advanced figurehead

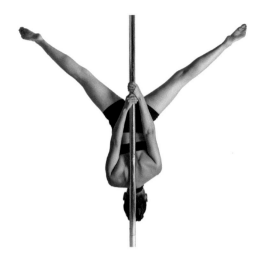

INVERTED PENCIL V

Points of support: Upper back and hands

Main focus: Assume a layback crossed ankle position. Keep the thighs adducted and the glutes contracted. Using a two-handed iguana grip, carefully slide the body down while maintaining a leg grip. Position the glutes below hand level with the arms fully extended and foot flexed to provide a secure grip on the pole. Release the ankle grip and move the legs off the pole, maintaining body alignment. When confident, fully abduct the legs.

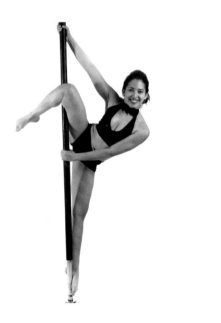

CUPID SUPPORTED

Points of support: Foot plantar, thigh, and back of knee

Main focus: Begin with a side climb. Hook the back of the knee around the pole, lowering the hips to achieve contact between the inner thigh and the pole. When confident, support and slide the far foot's plantar. Secure this position by keeping the hips forward and a strong hand grip on the pole.

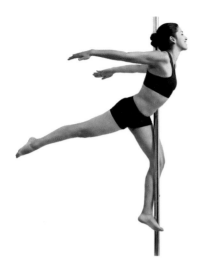

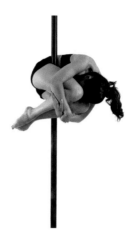

DART

Points of support: Underarm, flank, and shin

Main focus: Begin with an aerial leg hold position. Lean the upper body to one side and forward to anchor the pole under the near arm. When confident, extend the front leg backward while maintaining elbow extension. Grasp the pole with a near armpit hold.

TUCK DROP

Points of support: Thighs and flank

Main focus: Begin with a basic climb. Keep the knees flexed at the hip and the thighs adducted and strongly pressed to the pole. Lean the upper body to one side and tuck forward to knee level. Maintain the position while bringing the chest and trunk into contact with the thighs. Embrace the shins to secure the position. When confident, slightly abduct the thighs to slide down the pole. Rapidly adduct the thighs when approaching the ground.

SPACEFLIGHT

Points of support: Flank, leg, and hand

Main focus: Begin with a frontal pole sit and bring the knees toward the chest. Use the inner arm to embrace inner shin to grip the pole. When confident, extend the opposite leg backward. Maintain body alignment.

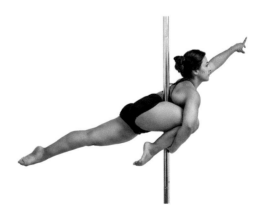

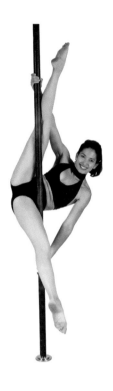

SIDE V

Points of support: Hands, groin, hamstring, and back of knee

Main focus: Begin with a side climb. Grasp the pole using a two-handed full bracket split grip. Take the far leg backward while maintaining support with the back of the knee. When confident, abduct the thighs and maintain near groin support on pole.

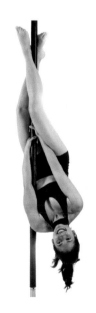

INVERSION LEG HOLD

Points of support: Hands and flank

Main focus: Maintain shoulder stability and grasp the pole with a strong hold grip. Support the inner hip on the pole. Engage the core muscles and invert the body, keeping the knees extended and the legs abducted. When confident, adduct the legs strongly on the pole. Use the ankles, calves, and shins to grip the pole.

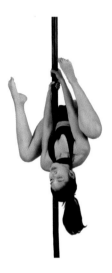

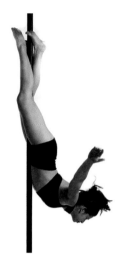

INVERSION LEGS TUCKED

Points of support: Hands and flank

Main focus: Maintain shoulder stability and grasp the pole with a strong hold grip. Support the inner hip on the pole. Engage the core muscles and bring the flexed knees to the chest. Invert the body and hold the position.

INVERTED CRUCIFIX

Points of support: Legs.

Main focus: Maintain shoulder stability and grasp the pole with a strong hold grip. Support the inner hip on the pole. Engage the core muscles and invert body, keeping the knees extended and the legs abducted. Adduct the legs strongly to the pole. When confident, release the hand grip, keeping pole at a midline position with chest and back extension. Ensure that the ankles, calves, and shins are gripping the pole.

INVERSION LEGS EXTENDED

Points of support: Hands and flank

Main focus: Maintain shoulder stability and grasp the pole with a strong hold grip. Support the inner hip on the pole. Engage the core muscles and invert the body, maintaining the knee extension and leg abduction.

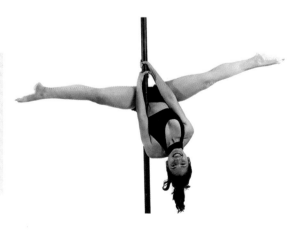

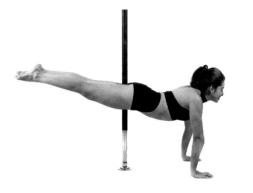

HORIZONTAL DISMOUNT

Points of support: Hands and thighs

Main focus: Begin in an inverted crucifix position. Gradually slide both legs down the pole to stabilize the hands on the ground. Take the hands forward while lowering the legs, keeping the body aligned and in the horizontal plane. Maintain thigh adduction.

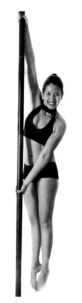

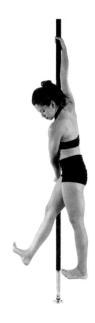

PENCIL FULL BRACKET SPLIT GRIP

Points of support: Hands

Main focus: Keeping an upright posture and shoulder stability, begin the exercise with a basic climb. Grasp the pole using a two-handed full bracket split grip. The hamstrings and glutes are fully contracted. Maintain a body position facing sideways to the pole and ankles in contact with each other.

AIR WALK

Points of support: Hands

Main focus: Keeping an upright posture and shoulder stability, begin the exercise with a basic climb using a two-handed full bracket split grip. Fully contract the hamstrings and glutes. Maintain a body position facing sideways to the pole and ankles in contact with each other. When confident, alternately flex the near and far legs, simulating a walking movement around the pole.

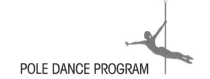

BASIC INVERTED SPLIT

Points of support: Hands and flank

Main focus: Maintain shoulder stability and grasp the pole using a strong hold grip. Support the inner hip on the pole. Engage the core muscles and invert the body, maintaining knee extension and leg abduction. Adduct the legs strongly on the pole and ensure that the ankles, calves, and shins are in contact with the pole. When confident, move into a leg split by lowering the near leg toward the ground and keeping the opposite ankle supported on the pole.

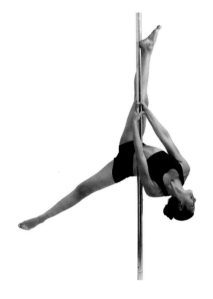

GEMINI ATTITUDE

Points of support: Flank, armpit, and back of knee

Main focus: Maintain shoulder stability and grasp the pole with a strong hold grip. Engage the abdominal muscles to perform a basic inversion. Hook the pole behind the far knee and flex the opposite leg. When confident, release the hand's grip and extend the arms backward. Grasp the pole with an underarm grip. Maintain an arched back and keep the inner hip supported on the pole.

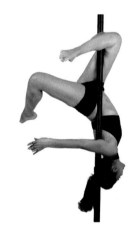

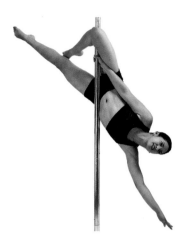

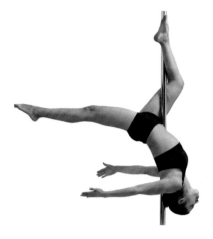

TOP-HANDED OUTSIDE KNEE HOOK

Points of support: Hand, abdomen, and back of knee

Main focus: Maintain shoulder stability and grasp the pole with a strong hold grip. Engage the abdominal muscles to perform a basic inversion. Hook the pole behind the far knee. When confident, release the inner hand's grip and extend the arm overhead. Maintain abdominal support on the pole. Extend the inner leg, maintaining proper body alignment.

SCORPION

Points of support: Flank, armpit, and back of knee

Main focus: Maintain shoulder stability and grasp the pole with a strong hold grip. Engage the abdominal muscles to perform a basic inversion. Hook the inner leg. Maintain an arched back and keep the inner hip supported on the pole. Extend the opposite leg. When confident, release the hand's grip and extend the arms backward. Use an underarm grip to grasp the pole.

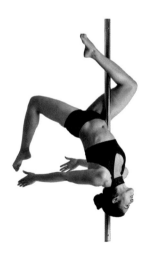

SCORPION ATTITUDE

Points of support: Flank, armpit, and back of knee

Main focus: Maintain shoulder stability and grasp the pole with a strong hold grip. Engage the abdominal muscles to perform a basic inversion. Hook the inner leg. Maintain an arched back and support the inner hip on the pole. Flex the opposite leg. When confident, release the hand's grip and extend the arms backward. Use an underarm grip to grasp the pole.

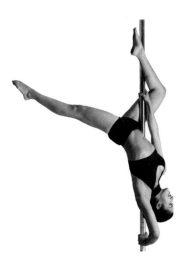

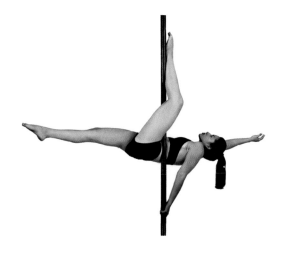

SCORPION HOLD (DRAGON)

Points of support: Hands, flank, and back of knee

Main focus: Maintain shoulder stability and grasp the pole with a strong hold grip. Engage the abdominal muscles to perform a basic inversion. Hook the inner leg. Maintain an arched back and support the inner hip on the pole. Extend the opposite leg. When confident, release the far hand's grip and extend backward overhead to hold the pole.

SCORPION FLATLINER

Points of support: Hand, flank, and leg

Main focus: Maintain shoulder stability and grasp the pole with a strong hold grip. Engage the abdominal muscles to perform a basic inversion. Hook the inner leg, extending the opposite one toward the ground. Maintain a near hand grip on the pole and support the hip. Extend the far arm overhead and maintain proper body alignment.

SCORPION (FOOT HOLD)

Points of support: Flank, armpit, and back of knee

Main focus: Maintain shoulder stability and grasp the pole using a strong hold grip. Engage the abdominal muscles to perform a basic inversion. Hook the inner leg. Maintain an arched back and support the inner hip on the pole. Flex the opposite knee. When confident, release the hand's grip and extend the arms backward, using an underarm grip. Hold the far foot with the inner hand. Back flexibility is required.

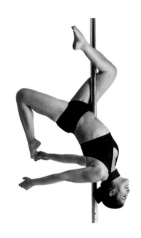

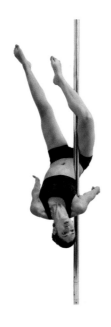
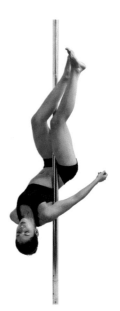

STATIC ELECTRIC LEG SWITCH

Points of support: Flank, armpit, leg, and back of knee

Main focus: Maintain shoulder stability and grasp the pole with a strong hold grip. Assume the Gemini position and rotate the near leg clockwise toward the pole and hook the releasing opposite leg's grip, fully extending it backward. The arms extend backward, ensuring an underarm grip. Maintain an arched back and an inner hip supported on the pole. Repeat.

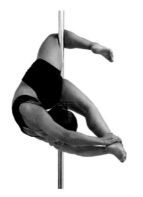

COCOON

Points of support: Back of knee

Main focus: Maintain shoulder stability and grasp the pole with a strong hold grip. Engage the abdominal muscles to perform a basic inversion. Hook the far leg. Maintain an arched back and an inner hip supported on the pole. Extend the opposite leg. When confident, release the hand's grip and extend the arms backward overhead to hold the far foot. Back flexibility is required.

BOW AND ARROW (ONE HAND)

Points of support: Foot dorsum, leg, and hands

Main focus: Assume a layback crossed ankle position. Keep the thighs adducted and the glutes contracted. Perform a two-handed iguana grip and carefully slide the body down, maintaining a leg grip. Position the glutes below hand level with the arms fully extended and the supported leg maintaining a flexed ankle grip. When confident, move the opposite leg forward and release one hand grip.

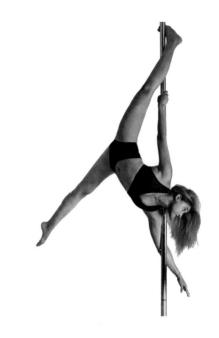

JASMINE

Points of support: Hand, groin, and back of knee

Main focus: Maintain shoulder stability and grasp the pole with a strong hold grip. Engage the abdominal muscles to perform a basic inversion. Hook the pole behind the far knee. When confident, support the inner hand on the pole and extend the opposite arm overhead. Maintain groin support on pole and extend the near leg while maintaining proper body alignment.

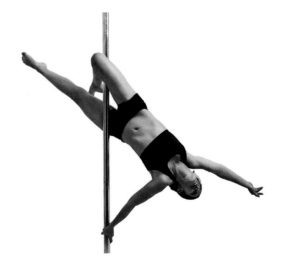

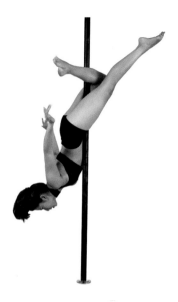

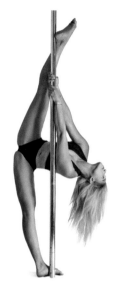

DRAGONFLY (INVERTED THIGH HOLD)

Points of support: Legs

Main focus: Begin in a Gemini position. When confident, rotate the body, keeping the pole in a midline position with the chest. Maintain back and near leg extension, strongly adducting the thighs to the pole.

SIDE POLE STRADDLE

Points of support: Hands and feet plantar

Main focus: Support the far foot on the pole. Maintain balance and grasp the pole with a baseball grip. Bend the upper body sideways, gradually lowering the hand's grip. When confident, raise the near leg and support the ankle on the pole, maintaining split legs.

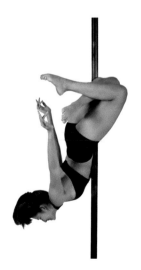

DRAGONFLY CROSSED

Points of support: Legs

Main focus: Begin in a Gemini position. When confident, rotate the body, bringing the pole to a midline position with chest. Flex the near leg and cross it over the opposite leg, strongly adducting the thighs to the pole. Maintain back extension.

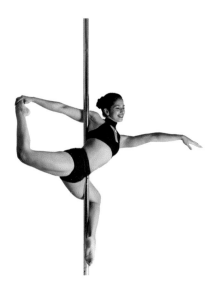

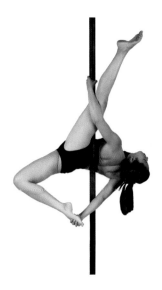

CAPEZIO

Points of support: Armpit, flank, and thigh

Main focus: Begin with an aerial ballerina spin. When confident, release the upper hand grip to lean back and anchor the pole under the armpit reaching backward to hold the foot. When confident, extend the lower leg, maintaining the lower hand's grip. Momentum technique is highly recommended.

ALLEGRA

Points of support: Flank, hand, and thigh

Main focus: Begin in a scorpion position. The near hand reaches up to hold the pole behind the near leg at knee level. Maintain grip and back extension. When confident, fully extend the near leg, flex the far knee, and reach to it with the far hand behind the pole. Back flexibility is required.

ALLEGRA SPLIT

Points of support: Flank, hand, and thigh

Main focus: Begin in a scorpion position. The near hand reaches up to hold the pole behind the near leg at knee level. Maintain grip and back extension. When confident, fully extend both legs.

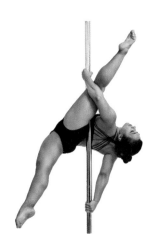

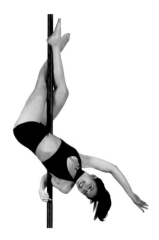

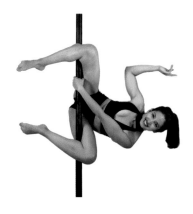

DORIS SPIN

Points of support: Flank, legs, and elbow

Main focus: Begin in a scorpion position. The near hand reaches up to hold the pole behind the near leg at knee level. Maintain grip and back extension. When confident, reach out to hook the far elbow around the pole. Bring the extended far leg and support it on the pole.

GENIE SUPPORTED

Points of support: Hands and back of knee

Main focus: Begin in a side V position. Grip the pole with the back of the near knee. When confident, take the far leg forward and hook the back of the knee on the pole. Maintain grip and upper-body alignment.

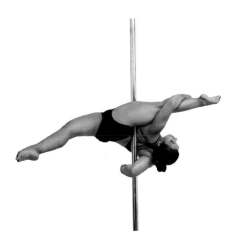

DORIS SPLIT

Points of support: Flank, legs, and elbow

Main focus: Begin in a scorpion position. The near hand reaches up to hold the pole behind the near leg at knee level. Maintain grip and back extension. When confident, reach out to hook the far elbow on the pole and support the hip on the far hand. Hold the near leg, bringing it toward the chest. Both legs remain extended in split position.

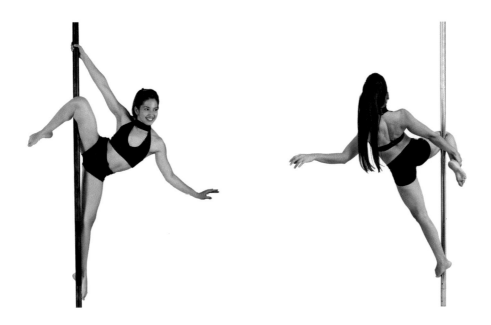

CUPID SIDE

Points of support: Foot plantar and back of knee

Main focus: Begin with a side climb. Grip the pole with the back of the knee. When confident, slide the far foot's plantar down. Secure the position by keeping the hips forward and a strong grip with the hand.

GENIE (NO HANDS)

Points of support: Hands and back of knee

Main focus: Begin in a side V position. Grasp the pole with the back of near knee. Take the far leg forward and hook the back of the knee on the pole. Keep the legs abducted and the hips forward, and strongly press the back of knees and calves on the pole. When confident, release hand grip and maintain upper-body alignment.

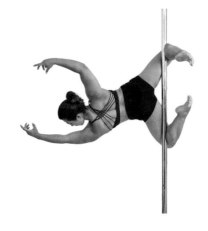

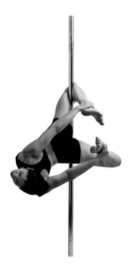

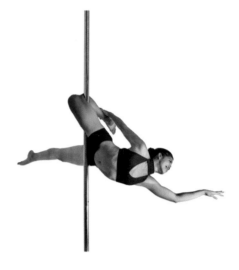

MARLEY

Points of support: Groin, thigh, and back of knee

Main focus: Begin in a side V position. Grasp the pole with the back of the knee. When confident, flex the far leg behind the pole and suspend the body, extending both arms backward to hold the ankles and create a back arch.

MARLEY FLATLINER

Points of support: Thigh and back of knee

Main focus: Begin in a side V position. Grasp the pole with the back of the knee. When confident, hold the near foot while keeping the hips forward. Extend the far leg behind the pole, suspending the body. Raise the far arm overhead. Support the groin on the pole and maintain body alignment.

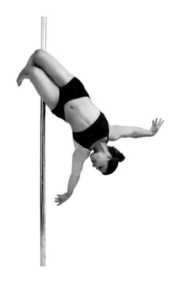

DOUBLE KNEE HOOK RELEASE

Points of support: Back of knees and hamstring

Main focus: Begin with a shoulder mount jackknife. When inverted, hook the back of the knees on the pole. Keep the hips leaned backward. Once the position is secured, release the hands, turning the upper body sideways to the pole.

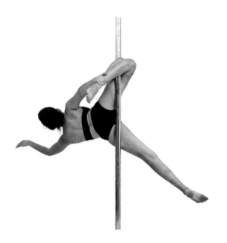

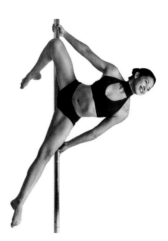

THE Q

Points of support: Hand, gluteal fold, and back of knee

Main focus: Begin in a side V position. Hook the back of the near knee around the pole. When confident, hold the near foot while keeping the hips forward. Fully extend the far leg to the front of the pole, suspending the body. Maintain far arm support on the pole until you feel confident to release the grip to raise the arm overhead. Ensure glute support on the pole.

DANGEROUS BIRD

Points of support: Back of knees and thighs

Main focus: Begin in a side V position. Hook the back of the near knee around the pole. When confident, extend the far leg to the front of the pole. Keep the hands equidistant from one another, the hips forward, and the legs adducted.

HIP HOLD PASSÉ

Points of support: Hands, groin, and thigh

Main focus: Begin with a two-handed half inverted grip. Engage the position by supporting the near groin on the pole and flexing the near knee toward the chest. When confident, extend the far leg backward and lift off the ground.

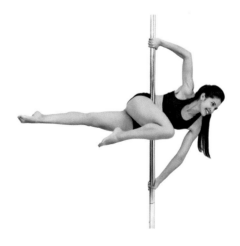

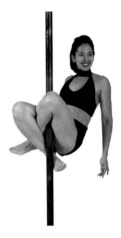

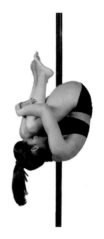

REMI SIT

Points of support: Back of the knees, thighs, and foot dorsum

Main focus: Begin in a pike sit position with a forearm grip. The forearm facilitates the body's distance to the pole. Flex the upper leg and hook the back of the knee around the pole. Flex the opposite leg over the upper leg at shin level and support the foot's dorsum on the pole. When confident, lean back, lowering hips to a sit position.

INVERTED THIGH HOLD TUCK

Points of support: Flank and thighs

Main focus: Begin in a Scorpion position. When confident, bring the near knee toward the chest and, subsequently, the far knee, keeping the thighs in contact with the pole. Secure the position by embracing the shins and pressing the knees toward the chest.

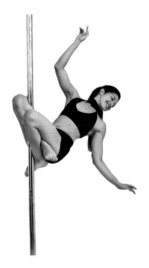

REMI SIT (LEG LOCK RELEASE)

Points of support: Back of the knees, thighs, and foot dorsum

Main focus: Begin in a Remi sit position. Grip the pole with the back of the knee and the foot's dorsum. When confident, lean back, releasing the hand's grip.

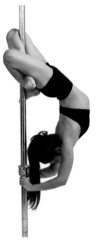

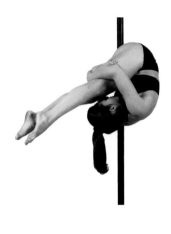

LOTUS BRIDGE (LEG LOCK BRIDGE)

Points of support: Back of the knees, thighs, and foot dorsum

Main focus: Begin in a Remi sit position. Grip the pole with the back of the knee and the foot's dorsum. Lean back, releasing the hand's grip and arch the back to reach an inverted two-handed double bridge arch.

INVERTED THIGH HOLD PIKE

Points of support: Flank and thighs

Main focus: Begin in a Scorpion position. Bring the near knee toward the chest and, subsequently, the far knee, ensuring contact between the thighs and the pole. When confident, fully extend and adduct the legs. Secure the position by embracing the hamstrings and pressing the knees toward the chest.

CHINESE POLE SIT

Points of support: Feet's planter, flank, and underarm

Main focus: Begin with a Chinese climb. Tilt the upper body sideways and forward to anchor the pole under the arm. When confident, abduct the near leg. Maintain the far foot dorsum support on the pole.

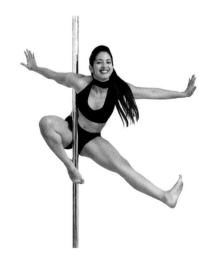

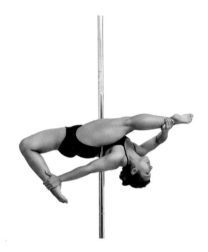

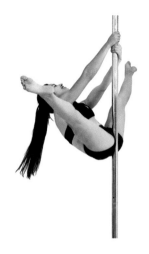

HALF JADE

Points of support: Flank, thighs, and armpit

Main focus: Begin in a Scorpion position, gripping the pole with the near leg. When confident bring the far leg toward the chest and embrace it. Extend the far leg. Grip the pole with the thigh and flank to the hold position.

JUMPING STRADDLE SPLIT

Points of support: Hands and gluteal fold

Main focus: Begin with a pike pole sit. Slightly turn the hip sideways, supporting the pole under the glute. Rapidly lower the hand's grip, bring the knees toward the chest and extend the legs while leaning the upper body backward.

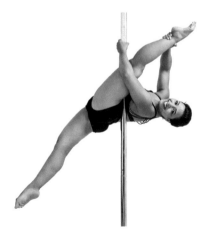

JADE VARIATION

Points of support: Flank, thighs, and armpit

Main focus: Begin in a Scorpion position, gripping the pole with the near leg. When confident, bring the near knee toward the chest and extend it, strongly pulling with the far hand. Flex the far leg and hold the ankle with the near hand. Grip the pole with the thigh, flank, and armpit to hold the position.

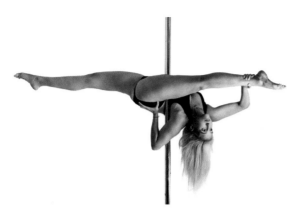

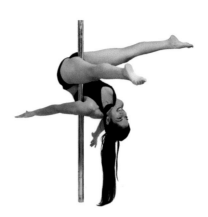

JADE

Points of support: Flank, thighs, and armpit

Main focus: Begin in a Scorpion position, gripping the pole with the near leg. When confident, support the hip on the near hand using an armpit grip. Bring the near knee toward the chest and extend it, strongly pulling with the far hand. The far leg remains fully extended. Grip the pole with the thigh and flank to hold the position. Extend the legs into a split.

HERCULES
(INVERTED HIP HOLD STRADDLE)

Points of support: Flank, thighs, and armpit

Main focus: Begin in a Scorpion position, gripping the pole with the near leg. Support the hip on the near hand using an armpit grip. Bring the near knee toward the chest and extend it. Then bring the far leg toward the chest, parallel to the opposite leg. When confident, release the hand support on the hip and extend the arms backward. Grasp the pole with the thigh, flank, and armpit to hold position. Extend the legs.

SUPERMAN

Points of support: Hand and thighs

Main focus: Begin in an extended leg inversion. Hook the back of the near knee above waist level and grasp the pole with a two-handed full bracket split grip. Extend the trunk in the horizontal plane and press the far leg against the pole. When confident, abduct the thighs, supporting the near groin on the pole. Rapidly turn the hips toward the ground, adducting the legs and releasing the lower hand grip. Remain in the horizontal plane with proper body alignment.

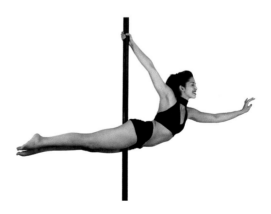

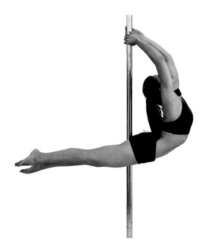

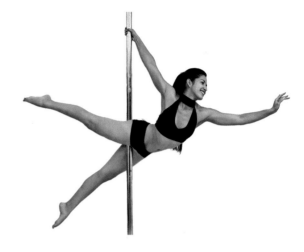

SUPERMAN CRESCENT

Points of support: Hands and thighs.

Main focus: Begin in a Superman position. Flex the upper elbow to approach the pole and assume a two-handed double bridge arch. Arch the back, pushing the chest down and fully extending the arms overhead. Keep the thighs adducted and elevate the legs.

SUPERMAN SCISSORS

Points of support: Hand and thighs

Main focus: Begin in a Superman position. Strongly adduct the thighs to the pole and keep the glutes contracted. When confident, move the legs vertically away from each other. Keep the thighs adducted and maintain a moderate back arch.

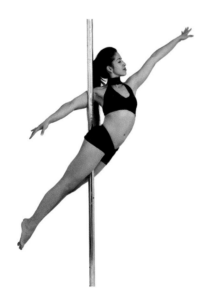

SUPERMAN (ARMPIT GRIP)

Points of support: Armpit and thighs

Main focus: Begin in a Superman position. Flex the elbows overhead to approach the pole and grasp it using a hook armpit grip. Press the arm toward the pole and keep the thighs adducted. Back flexibility is required.

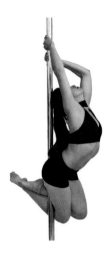

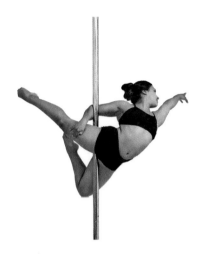

SEAHORSE

Points of support: Hand, tailbone, calves, and back of knee

Main focus: Begin in a Superman position. Strongly adduct the thighs to the pole. When confident, use a two-handed double bridge arch and rotate the right leg forward to hook the back of the knee around the pole. Flex both knees. Keep the thighs adducted and the back arched.

ANASTASIA

Points of support: Elbow pit, gluteal fold, and thigh

Main focus: Begin in a Superman position. Flex the elbows to approach the pole and hook one elbow around the pole, reaching out to hold the thigh. The opposite knee flexes, maintaining contact between the thigh and the pole. Back flexibility is required.

TITANIC

Points of support: Legs and tailbone

Main focus: Begin in a Superman position. Strongly adduct the thighs to the pole. When confident, extend the leg forward to support it on the pole. The opposite thigh remains adducted and elevated backward. Maintain back arch.

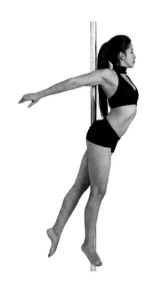

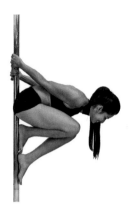

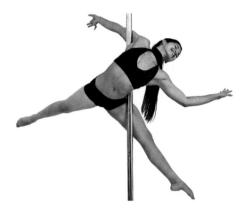

THINKER

Points of support: Hands, tailbone, and feet

Main focus: Begin in a Superman position. Strongly adduct the thighs to the pole and keep the glutes contracted. When confident, use a back grip with extended shoulders and elbows, while taking the legs forward. Maintain tailbone and plantar support on the pole.

STAR (FLYING BALLERINA)

Points of support: Armpit, flank, and thigh

Main focus: Begin with an aerial ballerina spin. When confident, release the upper hand grip to lean backward, anchoring the pole under the armpit while fully extending the arms and legs. Keep the near thigh in contact with the pole. Momentum technique is highly recommended.

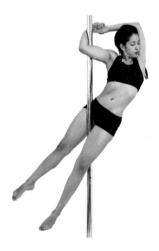

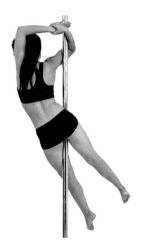

VORTEX

Points of support: Elbow pit, back of knee, and thighs

Main focus: Begin with a side climb variation. Fully extend the legs and lean forward to hook the near elbow around the pole. Maintain body extension throughout the exercise.

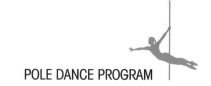

SUPERPAIN (NO HANDS SUPERMAN)

Points of support: Calves and thighs

Main focus: Begin in a Superman position. Flex the elbows overhead to approach the pole. Fully flex either knee and reach out to hold the foot's dorsum. Grasp the pole with a calf grip and back arch. Flex the opposite knee, keeping the thigh in contact with the pole. Back flexibility is required.

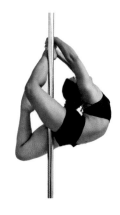

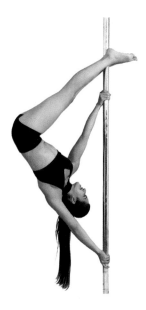

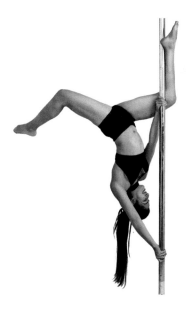

INVERTED D

Points of support: Hands and ankles

Main focus: Begin with an inversion leg hold. Extend one arm overhead and grasp the pole using a two-handed full bracket split grip or two-handed twisted grip. When confident, flex the hips, pushing the body away from the pole until it reaches ankle support. Keep the legs extended and maintain a centralized body position.

BUTTERFLY SPLIT GRIP

Points of support: Hands and leg

Main focus: Begin with an inversion leg hold. Extend one arm overhead to grasp the pole with a two-handed full bracket split grip. When confident, release the back leg's grip on the pole and extend backward. Flex the supported leg to secure the position. Keep the back of the knee, calf, and ankle in contact with the pole. Both knees remain flexed.

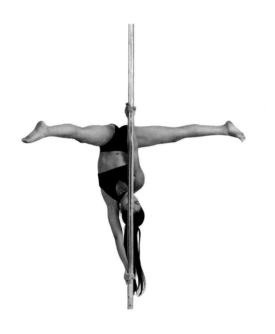

HANDSPRING

Points of support: Hands

Main focus: Begin with an inversion leg hold. Grasp the pole with a two-handed full bracket split grip. Flex the hips, pushing the body away from the pole until it reaches ankle support. When confident, flex the hips and abduct the thighs. Keep the knees fully extended and the pole between the thighs, facing the pubic bone. Maintain a centralized body position.

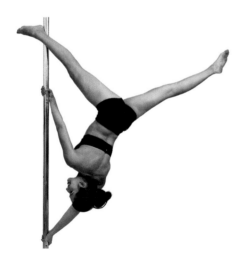

BUTTERFLY TWISTED GRIP (LEGS EXTENDED)

Points of support: Hands and ankle

Main focus: Begin with an inversion leg hold. Grasp the pole with a two-handed twisted grip. When confident, release the back leg's grip on the pole and extend it backward. Fully extend the supported leg until it reaches the ankle to secure the position.

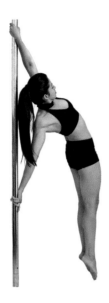

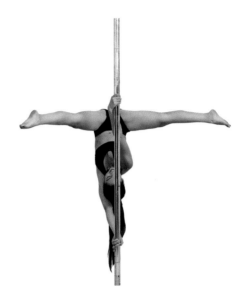

SPLIT GRIP HANG

Points of support: Hands

Main focus: Begin by grasping the pole with a two-handed twisted grip. Maintain shoulder stability. Turn the body to face away from the pole and extend the chest upward. The lower hand pushes the body away from the pole to safely lift off the ground. Maintain leg alignment.

TWISTED HANDSPRING

Points of support: Hands

Main focus: Begin with an inversion leg hold. Grasp the pole with a two-handed twisted grip. Flex the hips, pushing the body away from the pole until it reaches ankle support. When confident, flex the hips and abduct the thighs. Fully extend the knees and keep the pole between the thighs, facing the pubic bone. Maintain a centralized body position.

HANDSPRING STRADDLE CUP GRIP

Points of support: Hands

Main focus: Begin with an inversion leg hold. Grasp the pole with a two-handed true grip. Flex the hips, pushing the body away from the pole until it reaches ankle support. When confident, flex the hips and abduct the thighs. Fully extend the knees and keep the pole between the thighs, facing the pubic bone. Maintain a centralized body position.

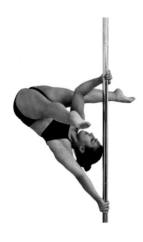

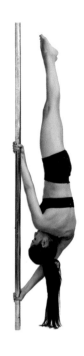

TWISTED HANDSPRING PENCIL

Points of support: Hands

Main focus: Begin with an inversion leg hold. Grasp the pole with a two-handed twisted grip. When confident, release the leg grip on the pole. To balance, the leg muscles must be fully contracted. Keep the knees extended and adducted. Align the body laterally to the pole.

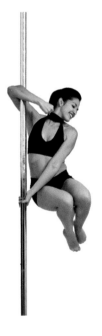

CHAIR (ELBOW GRIP)

Points of support: Hand and elbow

Main focus: Begin by grasping the pole with a two-handed elbow split grip. Hook the elbow above shoulder level and extend the far leg to procure momentum while leaning forward to spin. Flex both knees at hip level. Maintain a neutral pelvis. When confident, practice the exercise at a higher level on the pole.

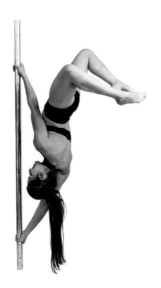

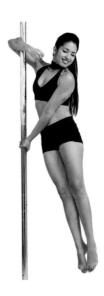

HANDSPRING FANG

Points of support: Hands

Main focus: Begin with an inversion leg hold. Grasp the pole with a two-handed full bracket split grip. When confident, release the leg grip on the pole, flexing both knees backward and assuming a fang leg position. To balance, the leg muscles must be fully contracted.

PENCIL (ELBOW GRIP)

Points of support: Hand and elbow.

Main focus: Begin by grasping the pole with a two-handed elbow split grip. Hook the elbow above shoulder level and extend the far leg to procure momentum while leaning forward to spin. Fully extend both knees, maintaining ankles in contact with each other. When confident, practice the exercise at a higher level on the pole.

CAROUSEL SPIN (ELBOW GRIP)

Points of support: Hand and elbow

Main focus: Begin by grasping the pole with a two-handed elbow split grip. Hook the elbow above shoulder level and extend the far leg to procure momentum while leaning forward to spin. Fully extend both knees, keeping ankles in contact with each other. When confident, attempt the exercise at a higher level on the pole.

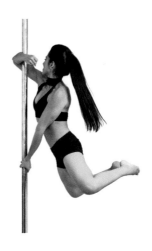

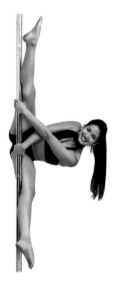

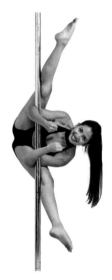

CROSS GRIP TULIP

Points of support: Hamstrings and hands

Main focus: Begin with a side climb. Grasp the pole with the back of the near leg's knee. With the far forearm supported on the pole, take the opposite leg forward, flexing the knee to maintain the back of knee grip. When confident, grasp the pole with a two-handed cross grip between the thighs, fully extending both knees and abducting the legs.

TULIP

Points of support: Back of knees and elbows

Main focus: Begin with a side climb. Grasp the pole with the back of the near leg's knee. With the far forearm supported on the pole, take the opposite leg forward, flexing the knee to maintain the back of knee grip. When confident, hook both elbows on the pole between the thighs, pressing strongly toward the chest, and fully extend both knees and abduct the legs.

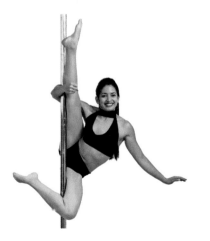

ALESIA HALF SPLIT

Points of support: Legs and elbow

Main focus: Begin with a side climb. Grasp the pole with the back of the near leg's knee and elbow, supporting the hamstrings on the pole. Take the opposite leg forward and flex the knee while maintaining the back of knee grip. When confident, fully extend the near knee parallel to the pole.

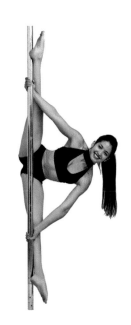

CROSSBOW (HANDS ON POLE)

Points of support: Hamstrings and hands

Main focus: Begin with a side climb. Grasp the pole with a two-handed split grip and hook the back of the near leg's knee over the near arm. Take the opposite leg forward, flexing the knee to maintain the back of knee grip. When confident, fully extend both knees and abduct the legs.

CUPID

Points of support: Foot plantar and back of knee

Main focus: Begin with the legs in an extended inversion. Hook the back of the far leg's knee on the pole, maintaining the hand grip. Support the near forearm on the pole while turning the body inward to support the near foot. The near knee remains flexed. When confident, extend the near knee and elevate the upper body, leaning sideways to the pole. Secure the position by keeping the hips forward.

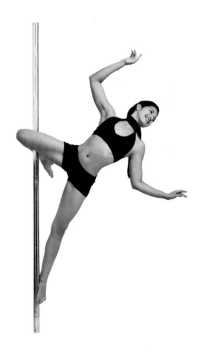

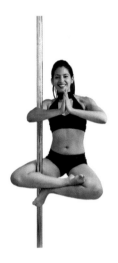

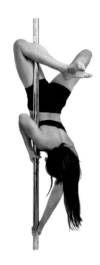

TEDDY BUDDHA

Points of support: Elbow, back of knee, and foot plantar

Main focus: Begin by flexing the hip forward to hook the back of the near leg's knee around the pole. Support the forearm on the pole to lift the body off the ground. When confident, raise the opposite leg to support the plantar on the pole. To secure this position, grip the pole with the elbow and lower the hips into a seated position.

BRASS MONKEY
(INVERTED BACK HOOK)

Points of support: Hands, underarm, and back of knee

Main focus: Begin in a layback crossed ankle position. Use the thighs to grip the pole and turn the upper body sideways to the pole, using a two-handed flag grip. When confident, strongly flex the near leg, securing the back of knee hook, and flex the opposite leg.

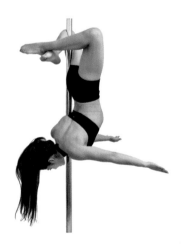

BRASS MONKEY VARIATION
(INVERTED BACK HOOK)

Points of support: Hands, underarm, and back of knee

Main focus: Begin in a layback crossed ankle position. Use the thighs to grip the pole and turn the upper body sideways to the pole, using a two-handed flag grip. Strongly flex the near leg, securing the back of knee hook, and flex the opposite leg. When confident, release both hands and extend the arms forward at shoulder level, grasping the pole with a near armpit grip.

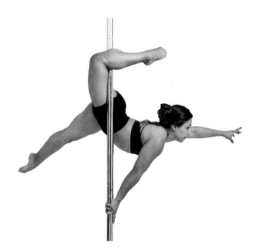

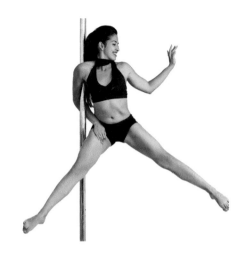

EROS

Points of support: Hands and legs

Main focus: Begin in a layback crossed ankle position. Use the thighs to grip the pole and turn the upper body sideways to the pole, using a two-handed flag grip. When confident, strongly flex the near leg to secure the back of knee hook and fully extend the opposite leg. The far hand pushes the pole away from the upper body with the near arm fully extended.

LIBELLULA VARIATION

Points of support: Underarm, elbow, and back of knee

Main focus: Begin with a side climb. Hook the near knee around the pole and tilt the upper body forward to anchor the pole under the near arm. Use an elbow hook to hold the inner thigh and fully extend both legs.

ADVANCED FIGUREHEAD

Points of support: Hands and thighs

Main focus: Begin in a Superman position. Flex the elbows to approach the pole and use a two-handed double bridge arch. Support the upper back on the pole, fully extending the arms over the head. Keep the thighs adducted, supporting the tailbone on the pole. When confident, elevate the ankles toward the glutes.

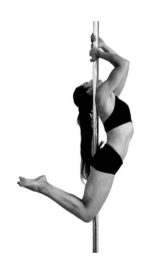

ADVANCED

The advanced level in the pole dance and fitness program contains the most essential pole stunts for achieving the highest levels of complexity in pole dance performance. The presentation of the stunts is analyzed according to each trick's characteristics and demands; in accordance with this pole dance and fitness guide, the previous pole dance program levels must be mastered in preparation for the execution of these advanced stunts. Technical guidelines suggested for each stunt must be considered, as well as safety measures to achieve an optimum performance.

Advanced pole dance tricks require strength, flexibility, and confidence. Advanced stunts are presented by a general classification of back flexibility, splits, and strength-based tricks. It is recommended to practice this chapter's exercises in order manner, aiming to perfect previous spins and tricks before moving on to learn the subsequent challenges.

ADVANCED PROGRAM

- Dakini
- Armpit hold hang (teddy passé)
- One-handed spin
- Armpit hold pike (teddy pike)
- Hawk
- Duchess (inverted hip hold passé)
- Vertical duchess (jade variation)
- Jade variation
- Standing split
- Meat hook
- Split grip leg through frontal split
- Frodo (cradle spin pike no hands)
- Side pole split
- Monkey split
- Daredevil
- Fish (Russian fish)
- Knee hold

- Broomstick
- Extreme brass monkey
- Bow and arrow (iguana shoulder grip)
- Forearm grip pencil inverted
- Janeiro
- Bow and arrow (no hands)
- Bow and arrow (elbow support)
- Russian layback
- Recliner variation
- Unicorn (Russian layback bridge)
- Iguana horizontal
- Iguana passé
- Fish hook
- Fallen star
- Back support split
- Marion Amber
- Jackknife (handspring twisted pike)

- Sneaky V
- Elbow grip butterfly
- Elbow grip pencil inverted
- Ayesha pike
- Ayesha fang
- Half flag straddle
- One arm flag
- Elbow mount straddle
- Flag grip pencil
- Toothbrush
- Back support plank (outside leg passé)
- Table top/back support plank
- Supported sailboat
- Iron X
- Iron flag (bottom leg passé)
- Iron X elbow grip
- Elbow hold passé
- Bat wing
- Elbow hold (lightning bolt)
- Libellula (dragonfly)
- Sword (elbow spin attitude)
- Elbow hang
- Dragon tail fang
- Reverse elbow hang (octopus)
- Eagle

- Dragon tail
- Bird of paradise (Up)
- Inverted bird of paradise
- Pegasus
- Swimmer forearm support
- Inverted Alesia half split
- Bendy split (bendy Philly)
- Armpit split (marchetti split)
- Marchenko (advanced rainbow)
- Hip hold split (machine gun)
- Reverse marchenko
- Chopstick
- Over split on pole
- Crossbow (spatchcock)
- Inverted front split body up
- Front split layback
- Inverted split
- Two-handed full bracket split
- Armpit hold split (Keem)
- Artamonova split
- Russian split hand release (flying K)
- Death lay
- Sign plus
- Icarus

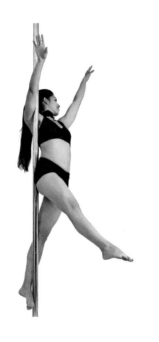

DAKINI

Points of support: Hip, armpit, calf, and foot dorsum

Main focus: Begin with an aerial leg hold or side climb. Take a strong hold arm position, supporting the inner hip and hamstring on the pole. Strongly hook the back of the inner leg's knee around the pole, maintaining the far foot's dorsum support. The pole should be anchored under the near arm. When confident, extend the near knee forward and raise both arms overhead.

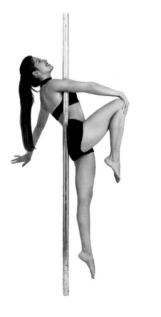

ARMPIT HOLD HANG (TEDDY PASSÉ)

Points of support: Hips, flank, and armpit

Main focus: Grasp the pole with an armpit grip and support the hip on the pole. Flex the far knee strongly and hold it with the near hand. The near leg remains fully extended and parallel to the pole. Use a secured armpit hold prior to flexing the far knee. When confident, release the far hand grip.

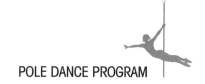

ONE-HANDED SPIN

Points of support: Hand

Main focus: Maintain an upright posture and shoulder stability. Begin with your preferred climb. Grasp the pole with a two-handed full bracket split grip or a two-handed split grip. The hamstrings are adducted and the glutes fully contracted. Preserve a body position sideways to the pole and ankles in contact with each other. When confident, release the legs and the far hand's grip on the pole, ensuring a near hand strong hold and elbow extension. Maintain shoulder stability, an upright position, and proper body alignment.

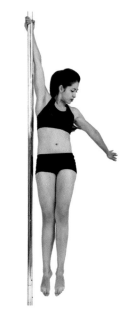

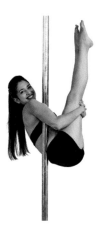

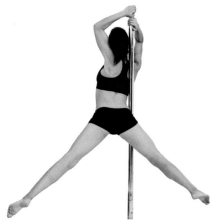

ARMPIT HOLD PIKE (TEDDY PIKE)

Points of support: Hips, flank, and armpit

Main focus: Grasp the pole with an armpit grip and support the hip on the pole. Flex both knees and embrace the thighs with both arms. When confident, extend both knees. Use a secured armpit hold prior to raising the legs.

HAWK

Points of support: Flank, hands, and thigh

Main focus: Begin in an aerial leg hold position. Lean forward, bringing the upper back into contact with the pole. Strongly hold the pole above the head with a two-handed cup grip with the elbows pointing out. When confident, release the legs to fully abduct and extend the knees.

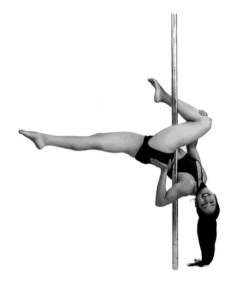

DUCHESS (INVERTED HIP HOLD PASSÉ)

Points of support: Flank, thigh, ankle, and armpit

Main focus: Begin in a scorpion position. Maintain a grip on the pole with the near leg. Support the hip on the near hand using an armpit grip and extend the far leg parallel to the ground. Use a thigh and flank grip to hold the position.

VERTICAL DUCHESS (JADE VARIATION)

Points of support: Flank, thigh, groin, and armpit

Main focus: Begin in a scorpion position with the near leg gripping the pole. Support the hip on the near hand using an armpit grip and extend the far leg up parallel to the pole. With the far hand, strongly pull the near knee toward the chest, using a thigh and flank grip to hold the position.

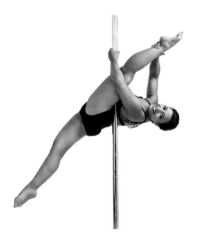

JADE VARIATION

Points of support: Flank, hand, and thigh

Main focus: Begin in a scorpion position. Reach the near hand up to hold the pole behind the near leg at knee level. The far hand pulls the near ankle, and both knees extend to a split position.

STANDING SPLIT

Points of support: Armpit, hips, and leg

Main focus: Begin in the soldier position. Support the far leg on the pole and grasp the pole using an armpit hook. When confident, bring the near leg toward the chest to reach the ankle. Keep the knee extended and pull toward the pole to assume a split position.

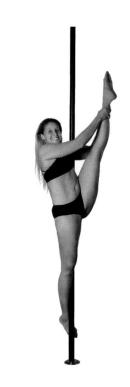

MEAT HOOK

Points of support: Hand, flank, and thigh

Main focus: Begin in the apprentice position. While spinning, support the near forearm on the pole and flex the near knee toward the chest. Bring the lower abdomen into full contact with the pole and bend the trunk sideways. When confident, release the upper hand grip.

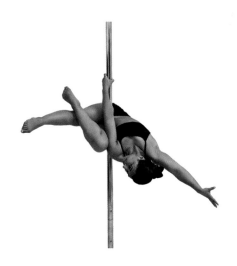

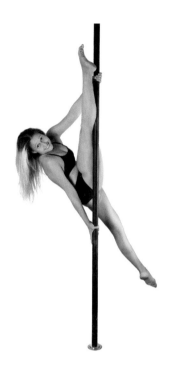

SPLIT GRIP LEG THROUGH FRONTAL SPLIT

Points of support: Hands and legs

Main focus: Begin in the brass monkey position. When confident, release both hands and contract the abdominal muscles to raise the upper body toward the legs. Reach the far hand to hold the pole above the leg with the near hand holding below the glutes and moderately twisting the trunk toward the near leg. Once the position is secure, extend both knees into a split position.

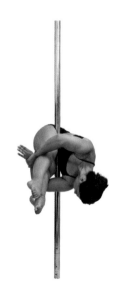

FRODO (CRADLE SPIN PIKE NO HANDS)

Points of support: Abdomen and thighs

Main focus: Begin in a tucked cradle spin position. When confident, release the lower hand grip to embrace the lower thigh, and release the upper hand grip to embrace the upper thigh. Strongly press the thighs toward the chest and extend the knees.

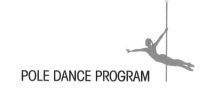

SIDE POLE SPLIT

Points of support: Hands and feet

Main focus: Use an overhead baseball grip with extended elbows throughout the exercise. Flex the knee and support the ball of the foot on the pole. Pull the body, gradually turning the knee toward the ground to support the sole of the foot on the pole. The opposite leg should be flexed and the hips aimed up. When confident, extend the upper leg and fully support the foot on the pole. Slide the feet until a comfortable split is achieved.

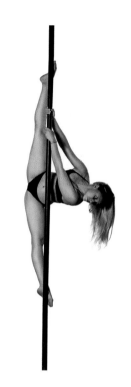

MONKEY SPLIT

Points of support: Hands and legs

Main focus: Begin in the brass monkey position. When confident, release both hands' grips and contract the abdominal muscles to raise the upper body toward the legs while the near hand reaches out to hold the pole and the far hand holds the pole below the glutes. The far foot remains flexed and hooked on the pole. When confident, extend the near knee to support the ankle on the pole while the far foot slides down to a leg split position.

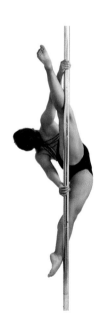

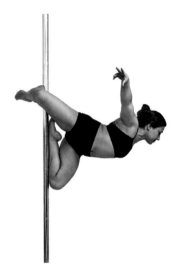

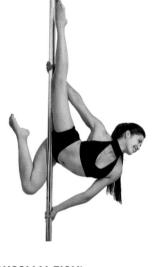

DAREDEVIL

Points of support: Legs

Main focus: Begin in a side hold position. Pull the body up to hold the pole above the hooked knee and to support the opposite knee on the pole. Keep the hips forward and knees flexed, securing the back of knee grip on the pole while twisting the trunk toward the ground. When confident, ensure far shin support, release the hands, and raise the upper body.

FISH (RUSSIAN FISH)

Points of support: Hands, legs, and foot dorsum

Main focus: Begin in a side hold position. Lower the hands' grip and arch the back, twisting the trunk toward the ground while extending one leg up to hook the foot on the pole. The opposite knee remains flexed and the thighs maintain contact with the pole.

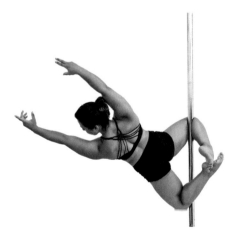

KNEE HOLD

Points of support: Legs

Main focus: Begin in a side hold position. Pull the body up to hold the pole above the hooked knee and to support the opposite knee on the pole. Cross the ankles, keeping the hips forward, and flex the knees, securing the back of knee grip on the pole. When confident, release the hands and lean the upper body sideways to the pole.

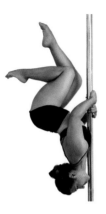

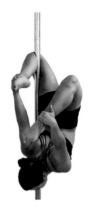

BROOMSTICK

Points of support: Chest and hands

Main focus: Begin with an inversion legs hold. Grasp the pole with a two-handed cup grip and fully support the chest on the pole. Release the legs' grip and keep the knees flexed. Hold the position.

EXTREME BRASS MONKEY

Points of support: Hands, underarm, and back of knee

Main focus: Begin in a layback crossed ankle position. Grip the pole with the thighs and turn the upper body sideways to the pole, taking a two-handed flag grip. Strongly flex the near leg, securing back of knee hook, and flex the opposite leg. When confident, release the hands and extend the arms backward to reach the feet. Hold the ankles while gripping the pole with the near armpit and back of knee grip.

BOW AND ARROW (IGUANA SHOULDER GRIP)

Points of support: Foot dorsum, hands, and shoulder

Main focus: Begin in a layback crossed ankle position. Keep the thighs adducted and the glutes contracted. Perform a two-handed iguana grip, carefully sliding the body down using a legs grip. Position the glutes below hand level with the arms fully extended while the supported leg maintains a flexed ankle grip. When confident, support either shoulder (trapezius) on the pole, fully extending the neck and either leg forward. Gradually slide the foot hook down while arching the back and taking the hips away from the pole.

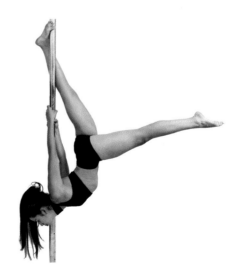

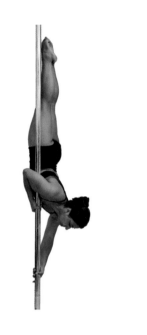

FOREARM GRIP PENCIL INVERTED

Points of support: Hands, underarm, glutes, and hamstring

Main focus: Begin in a layback crossed ankle position. Grip the pole with the thighs and turn the upper body sideways to the pole, using a two-handed flag grip. Strongly flex the near leg to secure the back of knee hook. When confident, extend both knees parallel to the pole. Hold the position.

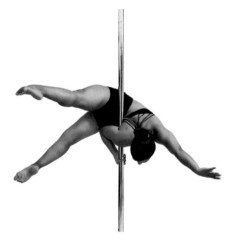

JANEIRO

Points of support: Hands and lower back

Main focus: Begin in the brass monkey position. Use far foot flexion to hook onto the pole and secure this position while lowering the near leg sideways toward the ground and supporting the lower back on the pole. When confident, release the far foot hook and bend the trunk to support the hip on the flexed arm. Release the opposite hand grip. Keep the back in contact with the pole throughout the exercise.

BOW AND ARROW (NO HANDS)

Points of support: Foot dorsum and legs

Main focus: Assume a layback crossed ankle position. Keep the thighs adducted and the glutes contracted. Perform a two-handed iguana grip, carefully sliding the body down and gripping the pole with the legs. Arms are fully extended. The supported leg uses a flexed ankle grip to secure the position. When confident, move the opposite leg backward while maintaining the thigh grip on the pole and the knee extension. Release the hands.

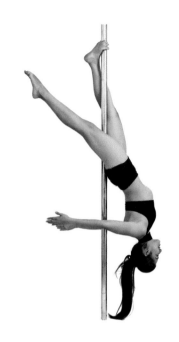

BOW AND ARROW (ELBOW SUPPORT)

Points of support: Foot dorsum, hands, forearm, and shoulder

Main focus: Assume a layback crossed ankle position. Perform a two-handed iguana grip, carefully sliding the body down and gripping the pole with the legs. Position the glutes below hand level with the arms fully extended and the supported leg maintaining a flexed ankle grip. When confident, support either shoulder (trapezius) on the pole, fully extending the neck, and release one hand's grip while holding the pole with forearm support. Gradually slide the foot hook down while extending the opposite leg forward. Arch the back and move the hips away from the pole.

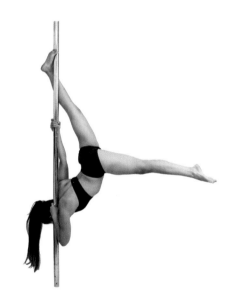

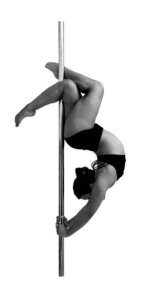

RUSSIAN LAYBACK

Points of support: Foot dorsum, back of knee, thigh, tailbone, and hands

Main focus: Begin in a genie supported position with the inner thigh supported on the pole using a back of knee hook and the hands. Cross the opposite leg over to hook the ankle with foot flexion on the pole. When confident, release the hands and lean backward to hold the pole above head level and ensure a two-handed double bridge arch. Keep the tailbone supported on the pole in a centralized position. Extend the feet plantar and hold the position.

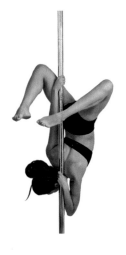

RECLINER VARIATION

Points of support: Hands, forearm, and shoulder

Main focus: Assume a layback crossed ankle position. Perform a two-handed iguana grip, carefully sliding the body down while gripping the pole with the legs. Position the glutes below hand level with the arms fully extended and the supported leg maintaining a flexed ankle grip. Support either shoulder (trapezius) on the pole, fully extending the neck, and release one hand's grip and hold the pole with forearm support. When confident, release the legs and flex both knees backward. Maintain toes contact with each other. Back flexibility is required.

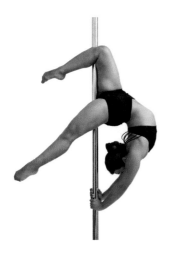

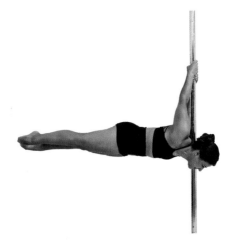

UNICORN (RUSSIAN LAYBACK BRIDGE)

Points of support: Foot dorsum, back of knee, thigh, tailbone, and hands

Main focus: Begin in a genie supported position with the inner thigh supported on the pole using a back of knee hook and the hands. When confident, extend the opposite leg, release the hands, and lean backwards to hold the pole above head level, ensuring a two-handed double bridge arch. Keep the tailbone supported on the pole in a centralized position.

IGUANA HORIZONTAL

Points of support: Hands and shoulder

Main focus: Assume a layback crossed ankle position. Keep the thighs adducted and the glutes contracted. Perform a two-handed iguana grip, carefully sliding the body down while gripping the pole with the legs. The arms are fully extended and the upper leg foot flexion is supported on the pole in a safe grip. When confident, release the legs off the pole, gradually lowering the body parallel to the ground.

IGUANA PASSÉ

Points of support: Back of knee and hamstring

Main focus: Begin in a double knee hook release position. When confident, extend the far knee parallel to the ground. The near knee remains strongly hooked to the pole to secure the position.

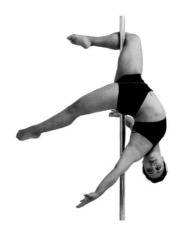

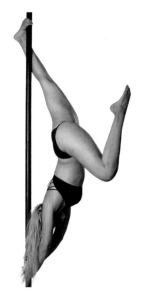

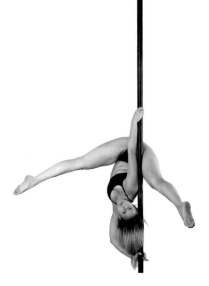

FISH HOOK

Points of support: Foot dorsum and hands

Main focus: Assume a bow and arrow position. Use a two-handed double bridge arch grip. Maintain foot flexion to secure the ankle grip on the pole. When confident, flex the opposite knee toward the chest and push the hips away from the pole. Hold the position.

FALLEN STAR

Points of support: Hands, thigh, and flank

Main focus: Begin in a scorpion position. While the near hand maintains its grip on the pole, extend the elbow and lean back to grasp the pole with the far hand grip above head level. When confident, extend the legs toward the chest in abduction. The near thigh remains in contact with the pole.

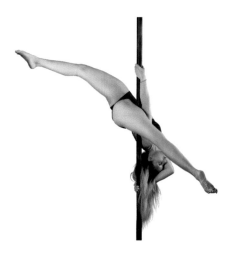

BACK SUPPORT SPLIT

Points of support: Hands, thigh, and flank

Main focus: Begin in a scorpion position. While the near hand maintains its grip on the pole, extend the elbow and lean back to grip the pole with the far hand grip above head level. When confident, fully extend the near leg toward the chest, keeping the thigh in contact with the pole. Extend the opposite leg backward toward the ground to assume a split position.

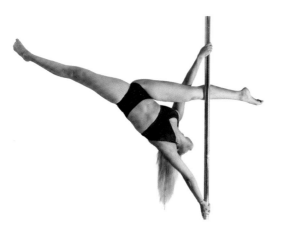

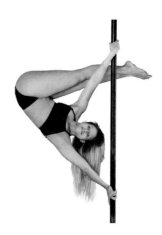

MARION AMBER

Points of support: Hands and leg

Main focus: Begin in an inversion with the legs extended. Assume an aerial side hold position, using the far hand to grip the pole above knee level. Flex the bottom elbow to strongly push the hips up until fully extended. Once the inverted position is achieved, lean the hips backward to fully extend both knees. Assume a split while keeping leg contact with the pole.

JACKKNIFE (HANDSPRING TWISTED PIKE)

Points of support: Hands

Main focus: Begin the exercise with an inversion legs hold. Use a two-handed twisted grip. Release the legs and fully contract their muscles to aid with balance. The knees remain fully extended and adducted. When confident, flex the hips to place the legs toward the back of the pole. Hold the position while maintaining leg alignment.

SNEAKY V

Points of support: Hands and leg

Main focus: Begin in a genie supported position. Bend the trunk sideways and toward the ground to support the far hand below knee level. Use the opposite hand to grip the pole between the legs. Hold the pole with the arms fully extended. When confident, release the back of knee hooks, leaning the hips forward and extending legs in abduction.

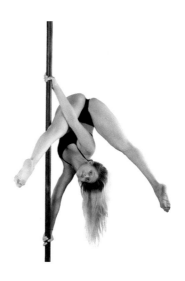

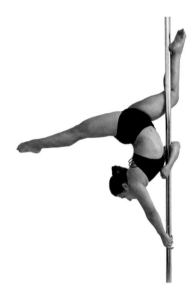

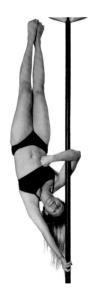

ELBOW GRIP BUTTERFLY

Points of support: Hands, arm, chest, and calf

Main focus: Begin with an inversion legs hold. Grasp the pole with a two-handed elbow split grip. Flex the hips and bring the chest toward the pole, keeping the upper elbow flexed and the lower arm extended. Lean the hips backward to support the calf on the pole and fully extend the opposite leg.

ELBOW GRIP PENCIL INVERTED

Points of support: Elbow and hand

Main focus: Begin with an inversion legs hold. Grasp the pole with a two-handed elbow split grip. When confident, release the legs and fully contract the leg muscles to aid with balance. Keep the knees extended and adducted. Maintain full-body alignment lateral to the pole.

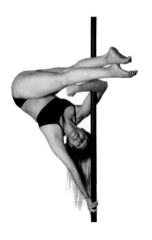

AYESHA PIKE

Points of support: Hands

Main focus: Begin with an inversion legs hold. Grasp the pole with a two-handed twisted grip. Release the legs and fully contract the leg muscles to aid with balance. When confident, flex the hips while keeping the knees fully extended and adducted. Hold the position.

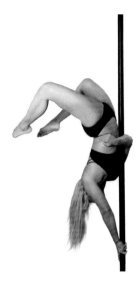

AYESHA FANG

Points of support: Hands, arm, chest, and abdomen

Main focus: Begin with an inversion legs hold. Grasp the pole with a two-handed elbow split grip. Bring the chest toward the pole, keeping the elbow flexed and the lower arm extended. When confident, release the legs and flex the knees backward.

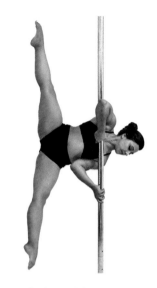

HALF FLAG STRADDLE

Points of support: Hands, arm, and chest

Main focus: Begin in a brass monkey position. Grasp the pole with a two-handed flag grip and support the flank on the flexed elbow. Release the legs and gradually lower the trunk sideways while keeping the thighs abducted and the knees extended to assume a split position lateral to the pole.

ONE ARM FLAG

Points of support: Hand, underarm, and flank

Main focus: Begin in an aerial leg hold position. Lean the upper body to one side and then forward. Use a two-handed flag grip to strongly anchor the pole under the near arm. When confident, extend both legs backward and the far arm forward. Maintain the armpit hold and continue to support the flank on the pole. Keep the far hand on the pole until you feel confident to release the grip.

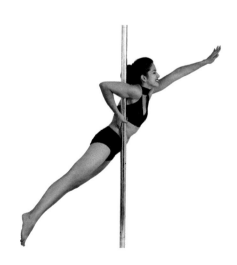

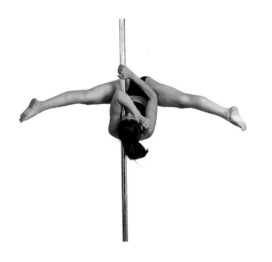

ELBOW MOUNT STRADDLE

Points of support: Hand, trapezius, and arm

Main focus: Comfortably support the shoulder (trapezius) on the pole and raise one arm overhead to flex and hook the elbow on the pole. The other hand grasps the pole with a cup grip. The shoulder remains supported. Contract the abdominal muscles, suspending the body from the pole. Both knees remain fully extended and the legs are adducted. Hold the position.

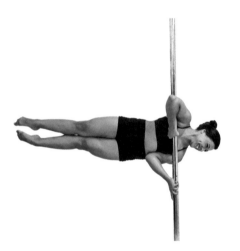

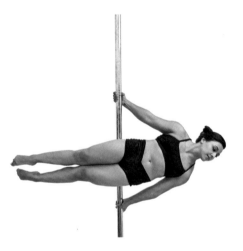

FLAG GRIP PENCIL

Points of support: Hands, underarm, and flank

Main focus: Grasp the pole with a two-handed flag grip. Support the far hip on the elbow to raise the legs off the ground. Keep the legs extended and adducted.

TOOTHBRUSH

Points of support: Hands and glutes

Main focus: Begin in a plank (hand on top) position. Raise one leg toward the chest to support it on the pole and hold it with both hands at knee level. Maintain glute support while twisting the trunk sideways to adduct the legs, supporting the lower hand below the lower leg. Arms should be equidistant to one another

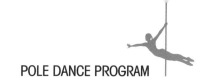

BACK SUPPORT PLANK (OUTSIDE LEG PASSÉ)

Points of support: Hands and flank

Main focus: Begin in a scorpion position. Grasp the pole with a near hand grip above the near leg support. The far hand holds the pole with two-handed baseball back support. When confident, release the near leg hook on the pole, maintaining knee flexion (thigh parallel to pole) and the far leg fully extended. Hold the position.

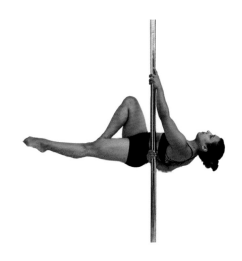

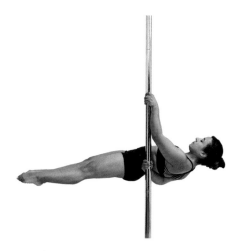

TABLE TOP/BACK SUPPORT PLANK

Points of support: Hands and flank

Main focus: Begin in a scorpion position. Grasp the pole with the near hand above the near leg support. The far hand holds the pole with a two-handed baseball back support. When confident, release the near leg hook on the pole to fully extend the legs.

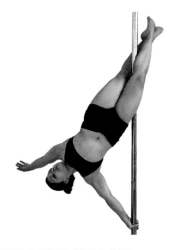

SUPPORTED SAILBOAT

Points of support: Hand, calf, and shins

Main focus: Begin in a brass monkey position. Extend the far leg to hook the flexed ankle on the pole. When confident, extend the near knee while supporting the calf and opposite shin on the pole. The near arm pushes the body sideways to the pole. Maintain body alignment.

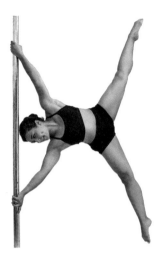

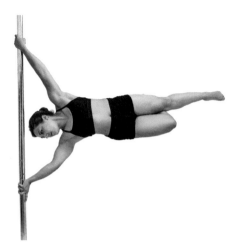

IRON X

Points of support: Hands

Main focus: Begin in a handspring position. Gradually lower the trunk sideways, keeping the hips forward and the legs abducted and fully extended. Maintain upper-body alignment and hold the position.

IRON FLAG (BOTTOM LEG PASSÉ)

Points of support: Hands

Main focus: Begin in a handspring position. Gradually lower the trunk sideways, keeping the hips forward and the legs adducted. Flex the lower knee and fully extend the upper knee. Remain in the horizontal plane, parallel to the ground. Maintain body alignment and hold the position.

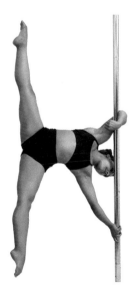

IRON X ELBOW GRIP

Points of support: Elbow and hand

Main focus: Begin in the Ayesha position, using a two-handed elbow split grip. When confident, push the hips forward, keeping the legs abducted while lowering the near leg toward the ground until a split position is achieved.

ELBOW HOLD PASSÉ

Points of support: Elbow, shoulders (trapezius), upper back, and hand

Main focus: Begin in a layback crossed ankle position. Reach out to hook one elbow on the pole. Support the lower shoulder (trapezius) on the pole using a one-hand down grip. Keep the chest in a lateral position while gradually lowering the trunk to release the leg grip on the pole. Hold the position.

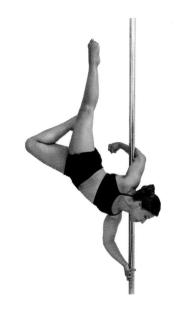

BAT WING

Points of support: Elbows and back

Main focus: Begin with a ballerina spin. Lower the trunk and rapidly hook the near elbow on the pole, use the far elbow to grasp the pole and support the upper back. Strongly flex both elbows to secure the grip while raising the trunk and abducting the legs to hold the thighs with the corresponding hands. Keep the split position parallel to the pole. Momentum technique is highly recommended.

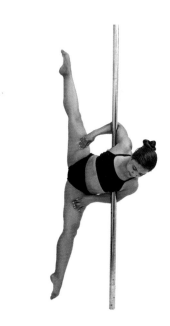

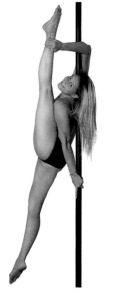

ELBOW HOLD (LIGHTNING BOLT)

Points of support: Elbow, upper back, shoulder, and hand

Main focus: Begin in a soldier position. Grip the pole with the legs and tilt the body forward, raising the near arm overhead to hook the elbow to the back of the pole. Support the shoulder. Contract the abdominal muscles to raise the legs toward the chest. The near hand holds the far ankle while lowering the into a split position. The far hand may remain supported on the pole or extended sideway.

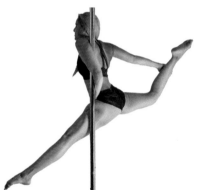

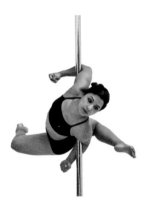

LIBELLULA (DRAGONFLY)

Points of support: Underarm, elbow, and back of knee

Main focus: Begin with an aerial half front hook. Hook the near knee around the pole and tilt the upper body forward to anchor the pole under the near arm. Hook the elbow around the pole to hold the inner thigh, and fully extend the near leg. When confident, extend the far arm backward to hold the far ankle.

SWORD (ELBOW SPIN ATTITUDE)

Points of support: Elbows and back

Main focus: Begin with a ballerina spin. Lower the trunk and rapidly hook the near elbow around the pole, then use the far elbow to hook around the pole and support the upper back on the pole. Strongly flex both elbows to secure grip, raising the trunk and legs in a double attitude position in the horizontal plane. Momentum technique is highly recommended.

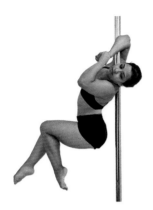

ELBOW HANG

Points of support: Elbow

Main focus: Begin in a Superman position. Flex the elbows over the head toward the pole and strongly flex the elbow to hook it around the pole. When confident, support the shoulder (trapezius) on the pole, hold the wrists and release the legs, flexing the knees toward the chest. Hold this position.

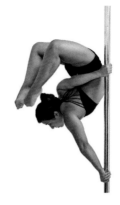

DRAGON TAIL FANG

Points of support: Hands and flank

Main focus: Begin in a Jasmine position. Keep the far hand on the pole and the elbow fully extended. Grasp the pole using a back support grip with the near hand. When confident, release the legs and flex both knees backward, maintaining a fang position.

REVERSE ELBOW HANG (OCTOPUS)

Points of support: Elbows, shoulder (trapezius), and upper back

Main focus: Begin in a layback crossed ankle position. Twist the trunk and grasp the pole using a two-handed double elbow. Gradually lower the trunk to release the legs and support the lower shoulder (trapezius) on the pole. Arch the back, separating the hips from the pole, and hold the legs in a fang position.

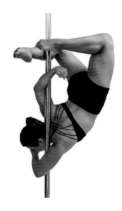

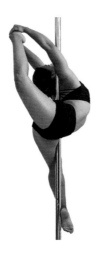

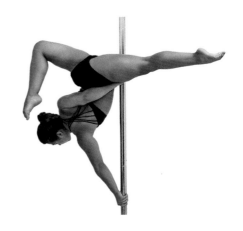

EAGLE

Points of support: Shoulder (trapezius), back, leg, and flank

Main focus: Begin in a ballerina position. Lean the upper body sideways toward the supported leg and grasp the pole with the far armpit. Twist the trunk, flexing the elbows overhead and reaching back to hold far foot. When confident, extend elbows and pull far leg backwards. Opposite leg maintains grip to the pole. Back flexibility is required.

DRAGON TAIL

Points of support: Hands, flank, and thigh

Main focus: Begin in a Jasmine position. The far hand maintains support on the pole and the elbow is fully extended. Grasp the pole with the near hand using a back support grip. When confident, extend the far leg forward and release the near leg, flexing the knee toward the back.

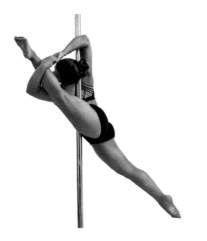

BIRD OF PARADISE (UP)

Points of support: Elbow, upper back, flank, and thigh

Main focus: Begin in a ballerina position. Lean the upper body sideways toward the supported leg and strongly hook the far elbow around the back of the pole. Release the near leg, extend it, and raise it toward the chest to hook the elbow at knee level. Hold hands to secure the position and bring the legs into a split position.

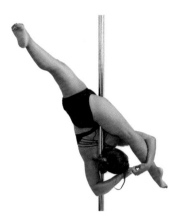

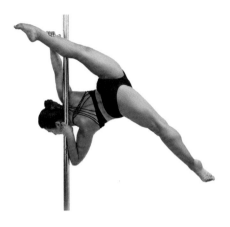

INVERTED BIRD OF PARADISE

Points of support: Elbow, upper back, flank, and thigh

Main focus: Begin in a Gemini position. Fully extend the near leg toward the chest and hold the ankle with the far hand. Strongly pull the leg, keeping it in contact with the flank and supporting the upper back on the pole. Hook the far elbow above head level and to the back of the pole, reaching out to hold hands at shin level to secure the position. When confident, release the far knee and extend the legs into a split position.

PEGASUS

Points of support: Elbows, shoulder (trapezius), forearm, shin, ankle, and upper back

Main focus: Begin in a layback crossed ankle position. Twist the trunk to grasp the pole with a two-handed archer elbow grip. Gradually lower the trunk to release one leg and support the lower shoulder (trapezius) on the pole. Arch the back, separating the hips from the pole. Keep one leg supported on the pole at shin level. When confident, release the upper hand holding the upper leg at ankle level. The opposite leg remains fully extended toward the ground.

SWIMMER FOREARM SUPPORT

Points of support: Elbows, shoulder (trapezius), forearm, and upper back

Main focus: Begin in a layback crossed ankle position. Twist the trunk to grasp the pole with a two-handed archer elbow grip. Gradually lower the trunk to release the legs from the pole and support the lower shoulder (trapezius) on the pole. Arch the back, separating the hips from the pole. The upper hand holds the foot and the opposite leg remains fully extended toward the ground.

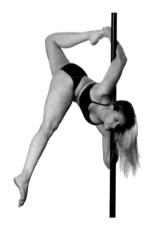

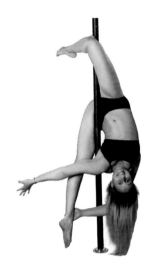

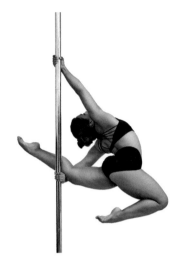

INVERTED ALESIA HALF SPLIT

Points of support: Thighs, back of knee, flank, and upper back

Main focus: Begin in a Gemini position. Lean backward, gripping the pole with a far knee hook. The near leg extends and approaches the upper body. The far hand releases its grip on the pole and holds the ankle, pulling the leg toward the pole. The opposite arm extends sideways.

BENDY SPLIT (BENDY PHILLY)

Points of support: Hands and shin

Main focus: Begin with a side climb. Lean forward and grasp the pole with the far hand, using a one-hand twisted grip. The near hand holds the pole with a basic grip below the supported knee. The elbows fully extend while arching the back and facing away from the pole. The far knee remains flexed and the supported leg fully extended.

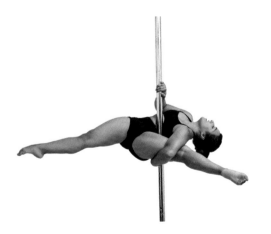

ARMPIT SPLIT (MARCHETTI SPLIT)

Points of support: Hands, flank, and thigh

Main focus: Begin with a side climb to a side hold position. Flex the far elbow to the hold pole with a basic grip between the legs and below glute level. The near hand moves to hold the pole between the legs, raising and releasing the near knee and fully extending it parallel to the ground. Move the legs into a split position in the horizontal plane.

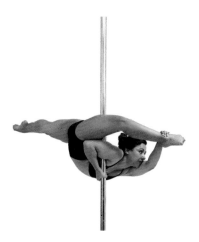

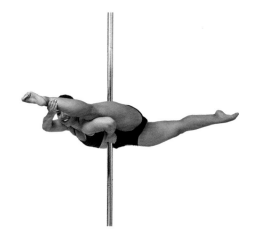

MARCHENKO (ADVANCED RAINBOW)

Points of support: Thigh, hand, arm, and flank

Main focus: Begin in a brass monkey position. Secure the grip by flexing the far foot on the pole while reaching back to hold the near with a two-handed flag grip. When confident, arch the back to pull the leg toward the head and extend the opposite leg parallel to the ground. Back flexibility is required.

HIP HOLD SPLIT (MACHINE GUN)

Points of support: Hands, flank, and thigh

Main focus: Assume a position facing sideways to the pole. Anchor the hips on the pole by supporting the near groin and flexing the knee upward. Lean the upper body forward to hold the pole in a one-hand down baseball grip with the elbow pointed out and hook the near leg over the near arm. When confident, extend both knees to bring the legs into a split position in the horizontal plane.

REVERSE MARCHENKO

Points of support: Glute, hand, and armpit

Main focus: Begin with a side climb into a soldier position. Hold the pole with the far hand while the near arm flexes back to reach the near foot. Keep the far foot flexed and hooked on the pole. Release the far hand and reach back to hold the near foot and adjust the armpit grip on the pole. When confident, arch the back and extend both legs. Back flexibility is required.

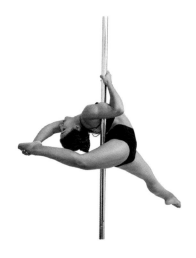

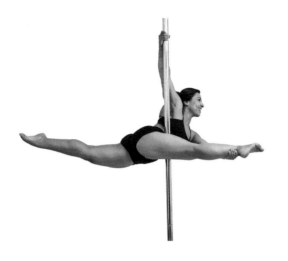

CHOPSTICK

Points of support: Hands, flank, and thigh

Main focus: Begin in a Peter Pan position. Fully extend the arms, maintaining the near hand grip on the pole. Lean sideways and forward to support the flank and thigh. Hold the upper leg at ankle or calf level, extending both knees to bring the legs into a split position on the horizontal plane.

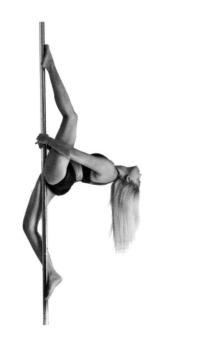

OVER SPLIT ON POLE

Points of support: Hands and legs

Main focus: Begin in a wrist sit position. Raise one leg toward the chest, supporting the foot on the pole as the opposite leg slides down the pole to bring the legs into a split position. Shift the hands to below knee level. If preferred, the knees may remain moderately flexed.

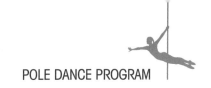

CROSSBOW (SPATCHCOCK)

Points of support: Calf, ankles, and elbows

Main focus: Assume an upright position, supporting the back on the pole. Grasp the pole with a two-handed reverse grab, supporting the shoulder (trapezius) on the pole. Contract the abdominal muscles to raise the leg toward the pole. Support the ankle on the pole while the opposite arm pushes the pelvis back to support the lower ankle on the pole. The upper body comes forward to support the back on the pole and the arms extend to secure the position.

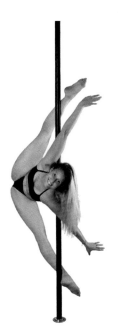

INVERTED FRONT SPLIT BODY UP

Points of support: Arm and legs

Main focus: Begin in a cupid supported position. Support the far foot and bring the full leg into contact with the pole. Lean the trunk toward the lower thigh, placing the hands in a centralized position on the pole. When confident, slide the upper leg on the pole until it is fully extended.

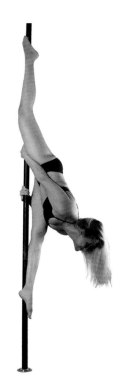

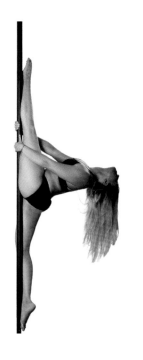

FRONT SPLIT LAYBACK

Points of support: Hands and legs

Main focus: Begin in a wrist sit position. Raise one leg toward the chest, supporting the foot on the pole, and side the opposite leg down the pole to a split position. Relocate the hands to knee level and fully extend both knees.

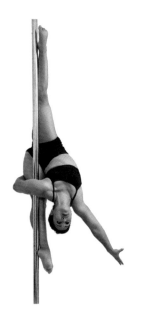

INVERTED SPLIT

Points of support: Arm and legs

Main focus: Begin in a cupid supported position. Support the far ankle, bringing the full leg into contact with the pole. Lean the trunk forward and hook the armpit on the pole. The arm embraces the leg and the near knee fully extends. Extend the arms sideways, maintaining an armpit grip.

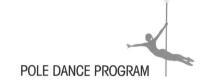

TWO-HANDED FULL BRACKET SPLIT

Points of support: Hands and feet

Main focus: Grasp the pole with a baseball grip with the extended elbows overhead. Flex the knee and support the ball of the foot on the pole. Pull the body, gradually turning the knee toward the ground to support the sole of the foot on the pole. The opposite leg is flexed and the hips aim up. When confident, extend the upper leg and fully support the foot on the pole. Using a full bracket split grip, slide the feet until a comfortable split position is achieved.

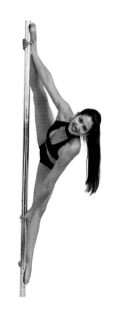

ARMPIT HOLD SPLIT (KEEM)

Points of support: Armpit and ankles

Main focus: Begin in an inversion, hooking the back of the far knee on the pole. Use the near forearm support to lift the body and take the near leg forward to support the ankle on the pole. Extend the arms to move the pelvis away, ensuring far ankle support. With the near elbow strongly hooked on the pole, extend the legs fully into a split position.

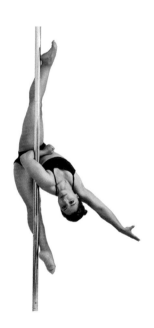

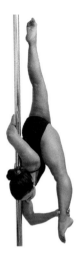

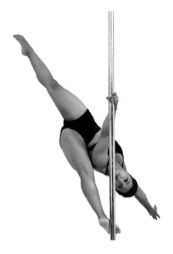

ARTAMONOVA SPLIT

Points of support: Elbow and shoulders (trapezius)

Main focus: Begin in a layback crossed ankle position. Reach out to hook one elbow on the pole, supporting both shoulders (trapezius). With the chest in a lateral position, gradually lower the trunk to release the legs. Lower the hand to hold the opposite ankle, assuming a split position lateral to the pole and extending the upper leg.

RUSSIAN SPLIT HAND RELEASE (FLYING K)

Points of support: Hand and foot

Main focus: Grasp the pole using a baseball grip with the elbows extended overhead. Flex the knee and support the ball of the foot on the pole. Pull the body, gradually turning the knee toward the ground to support the sole of the foot on the pole. The opposite leg is flexed and the hips aim up. When confident, release the far hand and extend both knees into a split position.

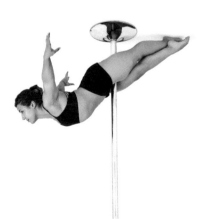

DEATH LAY

Points of support: Thighs and feet

Main focus: Begin by climbing the pole to the highest level to perform the harp, Superman, or advanced figurehead stunt. Making sure there is enough space between you and the ceiling, support the shoulder (trapezius) on the pole, using a two-handed cup grip. Contract the abdominal muscles to rapidly suspend the body and raise the hips to bring the pelvis toward the pole. When inverted, adduct the thighs to the pole and support the feet on the ceiling, raising upper body into the horizontal plane.

SIGN PLUS

Points of support: Armpit and ankles

Main focus: Begin with an inversion, hooking the back of the far knee on the pole. Use the near forearm to lift the body and bring the near leg forward to support the ankle on the pole. Extend the arms to move the pelvis away, using far ankle support. Hook the near armpit on the pole and fully extend the legs into a split position.

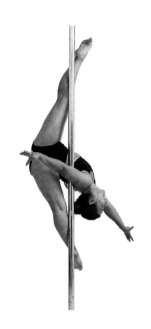

ICARUS

Points of support: Neck, upper back, and back of knee

Main focus: Begin with a reverse grab pencil spin. Using the hands to grip the pole, support the back on the pole. Lean the hips backwards and hook the back of the near leg's knee around the pole, maintaining the far hand's grip. When confident, release the near hand and lean head back, bringing the neck contact into with the pole. Release the far hand and extend the arms. The opposite leg remains extended sideways.

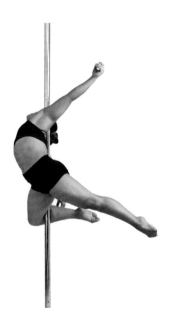

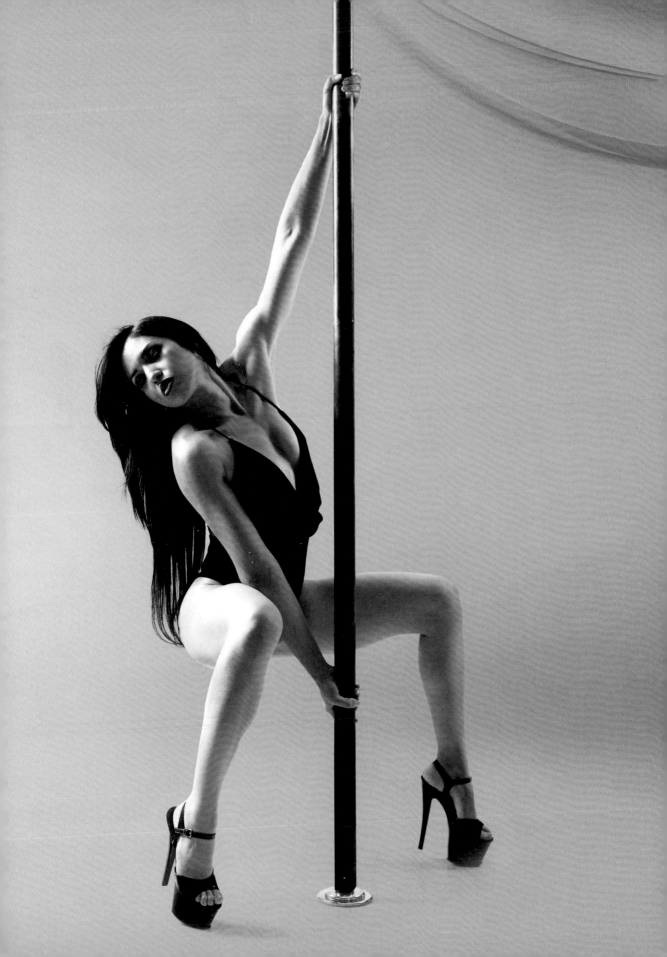

CHAPTER 10
COMBINATIONS

CHAPTER 10
COMBINATIONS

This section of the pole dance and fitness guide offers challengers a variety of movement combinations and tricks to perform to improve their physical endurance and resistance, as well as to develop artistic expression and fluency of the different movements. During the learning process, performers may freely incorporate different transitional movements, handstands, shoulder mounts, and climbs to embellish the pole dance routines. When choreographing a routine, it is recommended to select the most appropriate tricks based on the performer's confidence and fluency, and use the starting and ending positions of each stunt to select transitions from one pose to the next, as well as incorporating grounded transitions (floor work) and other movements that fit the music selected. Dividing the songs into sections to aid in memorizing the movements is highly recommended, choosing specific parts of the song in which certain tricks or movements will be performed. Writing down the movements and tricks selected during the choreography process has proven to be very useful, along with videoing your practice to evaluate the progress and identify possible strong and weak points of the performance to make the appropriate corrections and modifications. The most important aspect to consider is the challenger's artistic expression and emotionality while performing a pole dance routine; free expression and enjoyment are fundamental to achieving a graceful routine.

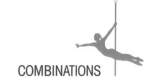

BASIC 1

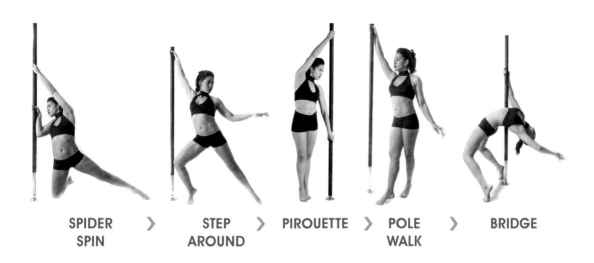

SPIDER SPIN > STEP AROUND > PIROUETTE > POLE WALK > BRIDGE

BASIC 2

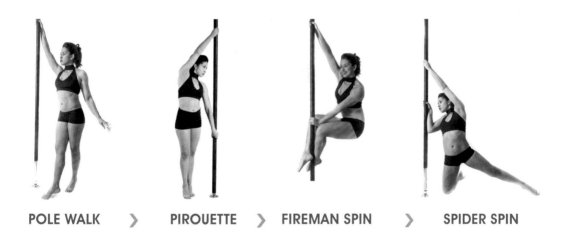

POLE WALK > PIROUETTE > FIREMAN SPIN > SPIDER SPIN

BASIC 3

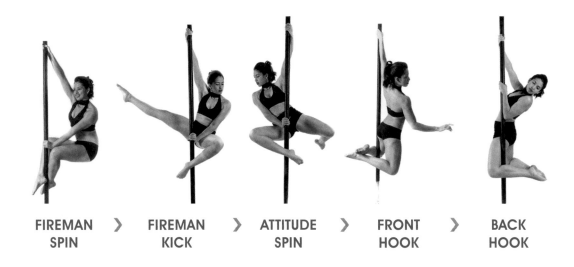

FIREMAN SPIN 〉 FIREMAN KICK 〉 ATTITUDE SPIN 〉 FRONT HOOK 〉 BACK HOOK

BASIC 4

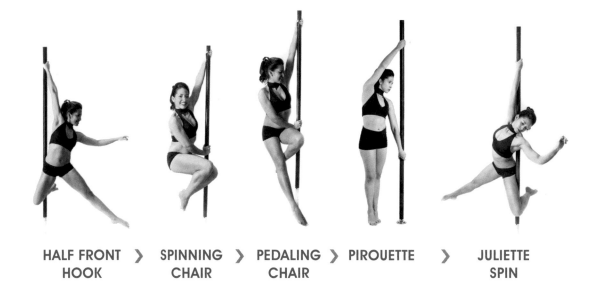

HALF FRONT HOOK 〉 SPINNING CHAIR 〉 PEDALING CHAIR 〉 PIROUETTE 〉 JULIETTE SPIN

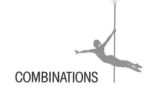

BASIC 5

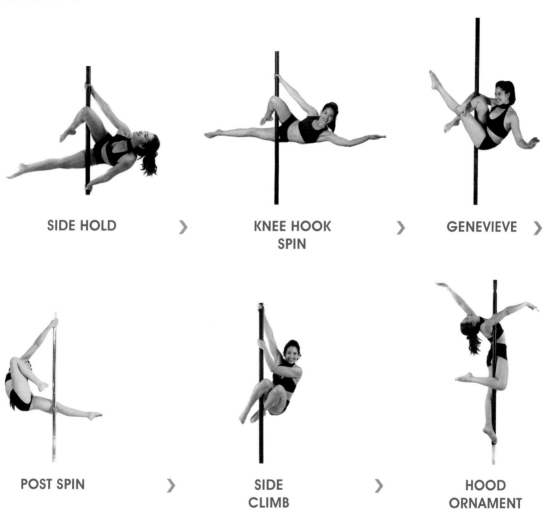

SIDE HOLD > KNEE HOOK SPIN > GENEVIEVE >

POST SPIN > SIDE CLIMB > HOOD ORNAMENT

BASIC 6

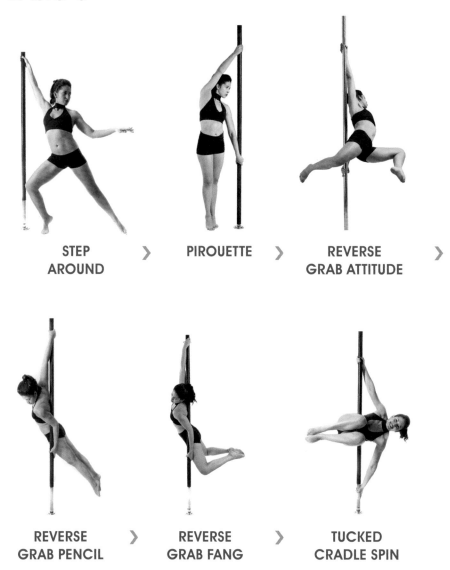

STEP
AROUND

PIROUETTE

REVERSE
GRAB ATTITUDE

REVERSE
GRAB PENCIL

REVERSE
GRAB FANG

TUCKED
CRADLE SPIN

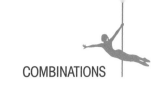

INTERMEDIATE 1

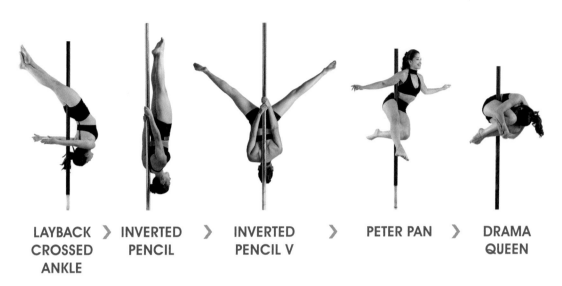

LAYBACK CROSSED ANKLE > INVERTED PENCIL > INVERTED PENCIL V > PETER PAN > DRAMA QUEEN

INTERMEDIATE 2

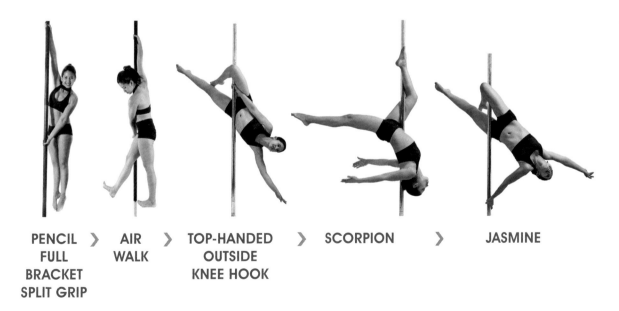

PENCIL FULL BRACKET SPLIT GRIP > AIR WALK > TOP-HANDED OUTSIDE KNEE HOOK > SCORPION > JASMINE

INTERMEDIATE 3

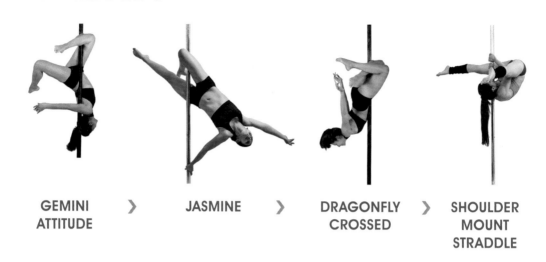

GEMINI
ATTITUDE

>

JASMINE

>

DRAGONFLY
CROSSED

>

SHOULDER
MOUNT
STRADDLE

INTERMEDIATE 4

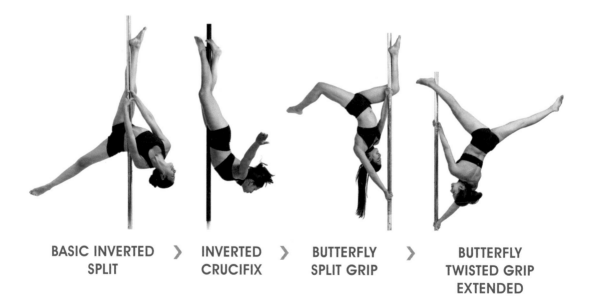

BASIC INVERTED
SPLIT

>

INVERTED
CRUCIFIX

>

BUTTERFLY
SPLIT GRIP

>

BUTTERFLY
TWISTED GRIP
EXTENDED

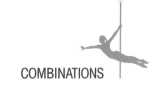

INTERMEDIATE 5

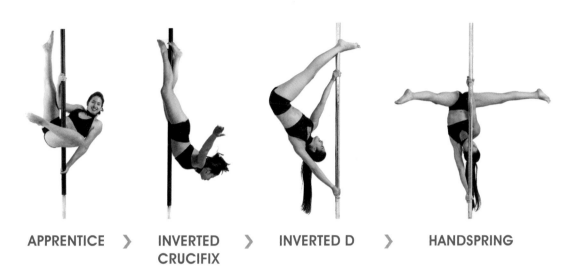

APPRENTICE ❯ **INVERTED CRUCIFIX** ❯ **INVERTED D** ❯ **HANDSPRING**

INTERMEDIATE 6

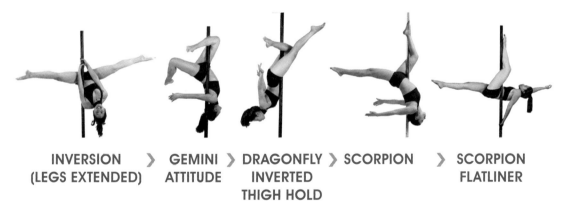

INVERSION (LEGS EXTENDED) ❯ **GEMINI ATTITUDE** ❯ **DRAGONFLY INVERTED THIGH HOLD** ❯ **SCORPION** ❯ **SCORPION FLATLINER**

ADVANCED 1

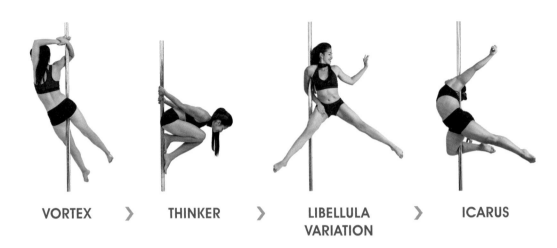

VORTEX > THINKER > LIBELLULA VARIATION > ICARUS

ADVANCED 2

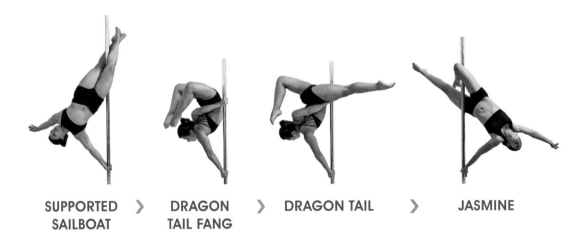

SUPPORTED SAILBOAT > DRAGON TAIL FANG > DRAGON TAIL > JASMINE

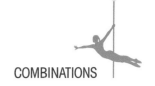
ADVANCED 3

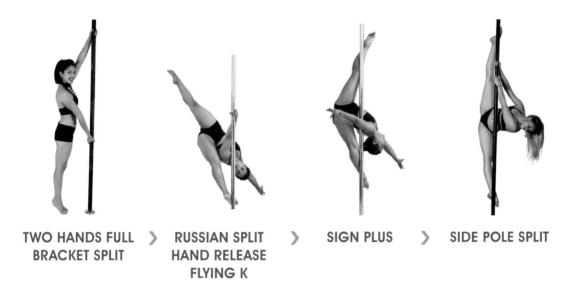

TWO HANDS FULL BRACKET SPLIT ❯ RUSSIAN SPLIT HAND RELEASE FLYING K ❯ SIGN PLUS ❯ SIDE POLE SPLIT

ADVANCED 4

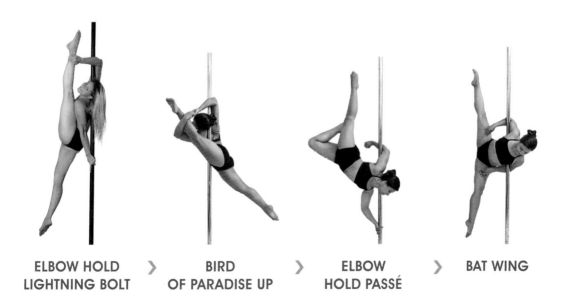

ELBOW HOLD LIGHTNING BOLT ❯ BIRD OF PARADISE UP ❯ ELBOW HOLD PASSÉ ❯ BAT WING

ADVANCED 5

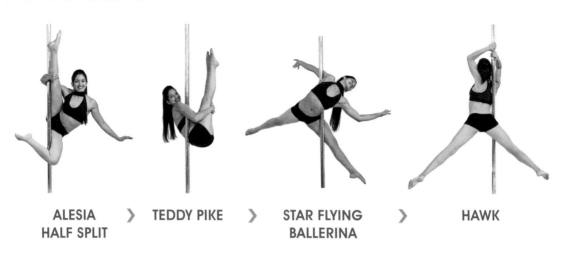

ALESIA
HALF SPLIT ❯ TEDDY PIKE ❯ STAR FLYING
BALLERINA ❯ HAWK

ADVANCED 6

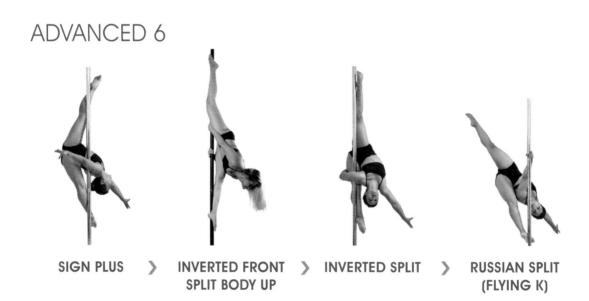

SIGN PLUS ❯ INVERTED FRONT
SPLIT BODY UP ❯ INVERTED SPLIT ❯ RUSSIAN SPLIT
(FLYING K)

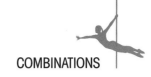

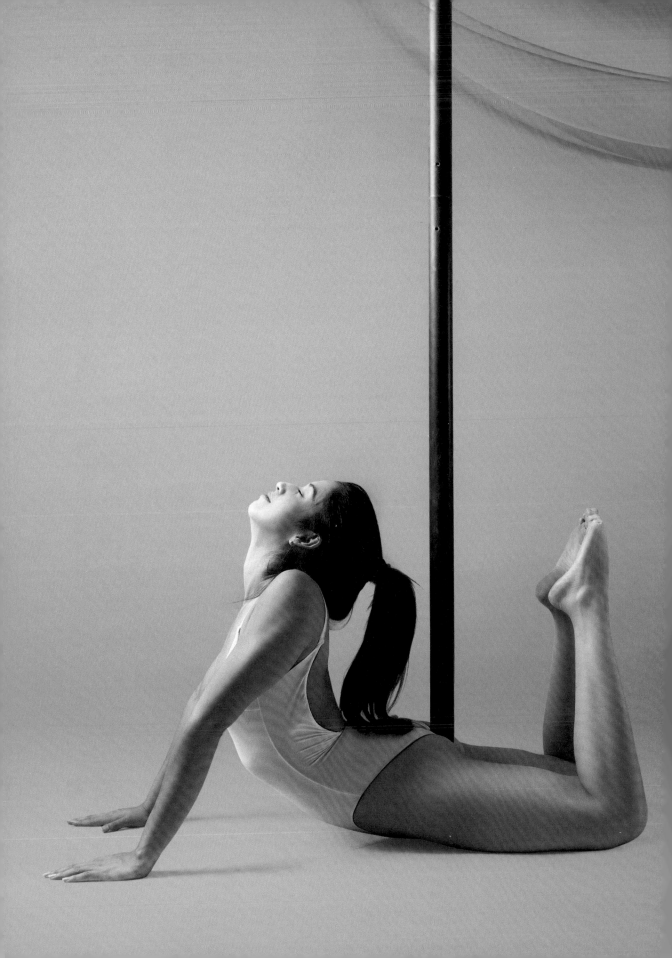

CHAPTER 11
POST WORKOUT STRETCHING

CHAPTER 11
POST WORKOUT STRETCHING

The post workout stretching section is dedicated to providing challengers with alternative exercises to be performed after pole training to improve circulation, stamina, and connective tissue reinforcement of the joints; to reduce muscular tension, soreness, and tendon injury probability; and to contribute to physical and mental relaxation, as well as flexibility, physical endurance, and range of motion, assuring an improved performance.

As in pre-workout stretches, all exercises must be performed progressively, entirely covering multiple body areas, while performing appropriate breathing techniques. Deep and regular breathing must be implemented into the exercise performance. To execute an optimal breathing technique, deeply inhale through the nose, hold the breath for 10-15 seconds, and exhale through the mouth. This is especially helpful when trying to increase a certain stretch. Contractions occur when a stretch exceeds the muscle's capacity, producing counterproductive effects. Considering breathing techniques will contribute to muscle capability, allowing them to tolerate further stretching movements.

After workout sessions, a relaxation and stretching period is highly recommended to gradually allow the heart rate and breathing frequency to return to a pre-exercise state, minimizing muscle pain and soreness after intense physical activities. A ten- to fifteen-minute full-body stretch routine may be sufficient, mobilizing major muscle groups with two or three repetitions on both sides of the body.

The pole dance and fitness guide provides general exercises that must be cautiously executed according to each performer's capabilities, individual characteristics, and conditions. Discomfort may be a common sensation while performing stretches, especially when intensity and complexity is augmented; however, pain is not a positive symptom. Aggressive stretches and drastic transitional movements reduce mobility control, increasing the likelihood of muscle strains and micro-tears. A regular review of the provided information according to specific muscle groups and each exercise performed will help challengers procure a proper alignment and prepare them for future accomplishments.

POST WORKOUT STRETCHES

- Grounded full forward fold
- Inverted pike stretch
- Lying flexion
- Single knee to chest stretch
- Low back crossover
- Lower back and hamstring stretch (A)
- Inverted contortion stretch
- Head-to-knee forward bend
- Bridge pose
- Cat/cow
- Lean back thigh stretch
- Kneeling lumbar flexion/child's pose
- Mild lower back stretch
- Hip flexors stretch
- Back extension
- Downward dog variation
- Sky reach
- Extended puppy pose variation
- Revolved triangle pose
- Downward dog
- Forward bend
- Intense side stretch pose
- Extended reverse stretch

- Back extension
- Finger flexion and extension
- Back and shoulders extension (A)
- Shoulder stretch (A)
- Hip flexors stretch (A)
- Hip flexors and hamstring stretch
- Back lateral flexion
- Rotational stretch
- Cross arm stretch
- Back and shoulders extension (B)
- Back and shoulders extension (C)
- Hip flexors stretch (B)
- Calf stretch
- Hamstring stretch (back to pole)
- Hip flexors stretch (C)
- Adductors stretch
- Split
- Shoulder stretch (B)
- Backbend stretch
- Back and shoulders extension (D)
- Deep backbend stretch
- Hamstring stretch

POST WORKOUT STRETCHES

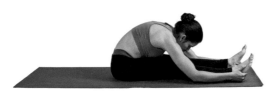

GROUNDED FULL FORWARD FOLD

Sit comfortably on the ground. Lean forward, keeping the knees extended knees and the upper body aligned. Hold the heels. Deeply inhale and try reaching further with each exhalation.

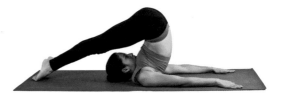

INVERTED PIKE STRETCH

Assume a supine position with the arms pronated. Raise the legs and hips. Engage the abdominal muscles and swing the fully extended legs backward. Keep the toes in contact with the ground.

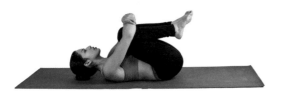

LYING FLEXION

Lie comfortably, maintaining full back support on the ground. Flex the knees to the chest. Hold the shins to maintain the position. Raise the head toward the knees to increase the stretch.

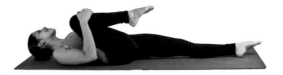

SINGLE KNEE TO CHEST STRETCH

Lie comfortably, maintaining full back support on the ground. Bring one knee toward the chest by holding the shin. Keep the opposite leg fully extended. Repeat on the other side.

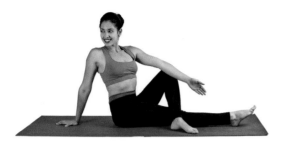

LOW BACK CROSSOVER

Sit comfortably on the ground with the left leg fully extended and the right knee crossed over it. Cross the left elbow over the right knee and gently press the knee over, twisting the torso to the right. Repeat exercise to the opposite direction.

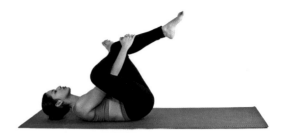

LOWER BACK AND HAMSTRING STRETCH (A)

Lie comfortably, maintaining full back support on the ground. With the right ankle crossed and supported over the left knee, place the right arm between the thighs and hold the left shin with both hands, pulling it toward the chest. Repeat on the opposite side.

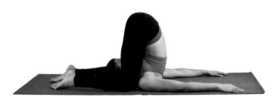

INVERTED CONTORTION STRETCH

Assume a supine position with the arms pronated. Raise the legs and hips. Engage the abdominal muscles and swing the fully extended legs backward. Keep the toes in contact with the ground. When confident, flex the knees while supporting the shins on the ground.

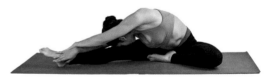

HEAD-TO-KNEE FORWARD BEND

Sit comfortably with the back extended. Abduct one leg sideways with the knee flexed and the heel toward the pubic bone. Abduct the opposite leg and fully extend it sideways. When confident, laterally shift the trunk toward the extended leg and raise the arm overhead. Repeat on the opposite side.

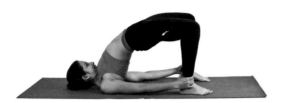

BRIDGE POSE

Assume a supine position. Raise pelvis, supporting your weight on the shoulder, and reach for the ankles. Keep the knees at a 90 degrees angle.

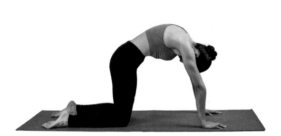 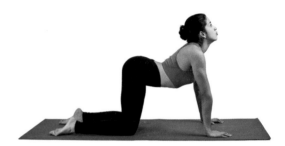

CAT/COW

Assume a quadruped position. For the cat position, arch the lower back down while extending the neck. For the cow position, arch the back up with neck flexion, tucking the chin in toward the sternum.

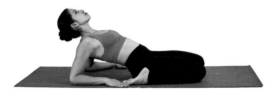 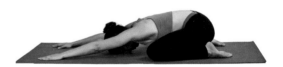

LEAN BACK THIGH STRETCH

Assume a prone position with the elbows bent to 90 degrees. With the forearms, palms, and knees in contact with the ground, abduct the thighs and lower the pelvis toward the ground.

KNEELING LUMBAR FLEXION/ CHILD'S POSE

Assume a quadruped position. Sit back, bringing the glutes into contact with the heels. Stretch both arms forward with the neck slightly flexed.

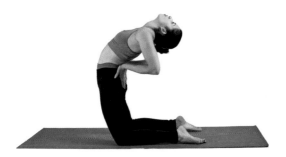

MILD LOWER BACK STRETCH

Place the hands on the posterior aspect of the pelvis. Slightly push the pelvis forward and extend the back.

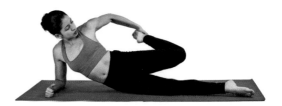

HIP FLEXORS STRETCH

Assume a position lying on your side. Keep the grounded leg extended and hold the opposite foot while flexing the knee and slightly pulling toward the glutes. Repeat on the opposite side.

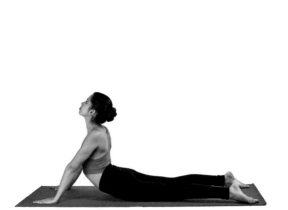

BACK EXTENSION

Assume a prone position with the hands supported, keeping the pelvis and lower legs in contact with the ground. Raise the upper back and extend while the neck and head remain in a neutral position.

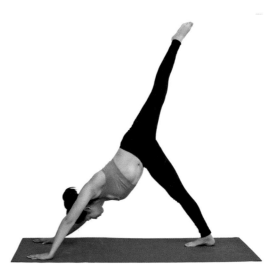

DOWNWARD DOG VARIATION

Assume a downward dog position. Slightly twist the hips inward and raise one fully extended leg while keeping the upper body aligned.

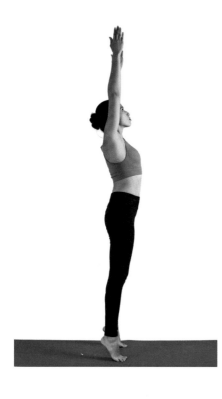

SKY REACH

Assume a standing position. Raise the arms overhead and reach up to extend the full body.

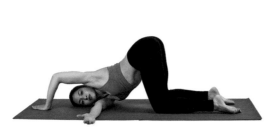

EXTENDED PUPPY POSE VARIATION

Assume a quadruped position with the hips and knees flexed to 90 degrees. Lower toward the ground and twist the trunk, keeping the arm extended and horizontally adducted. Repeat on opposite side.

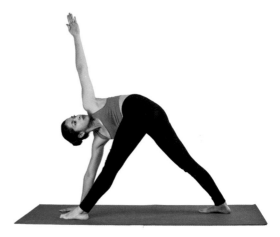

REVOLVED TRIANGLE POSE

Assume a standing position. Step one leg forward and lean the trunk toward the front leg. Bring the upper body into contact with the leg and reach the hands to the ground. When confident, raise one arm sideways to shoulder level. Repeat on the opposite side.

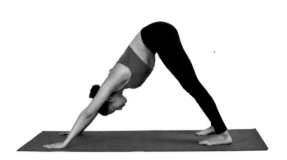

DOWNWARD DOG

Assume a kneeling lumbar flexion position. Fully support the feet and palms on the ground. Raise the hips, extending the back and maintaining upper-body alignment.

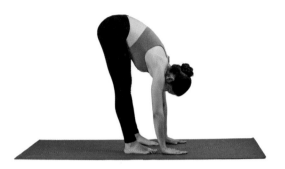

FORWARD BEND

Assume a standing position. Bend the trunk forward and reach down to place the palms on the ground.

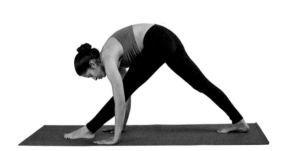

INTENSE SIDE STRETCH POSE

Assume a standing position. Step one leg forward and lean the trunk toward the front leg. Bring the upper body into contact with the leg and reach down to bring the hands to the ground.

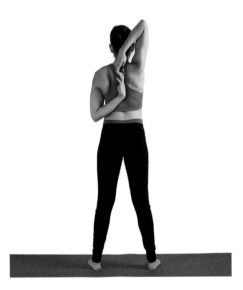

EXTENDED REVERSE STRETCH

Raise the right arm overhead and to the back of the neck. Flex the left arm behind the trunk. Interlock the fingers and slightly pull one another.

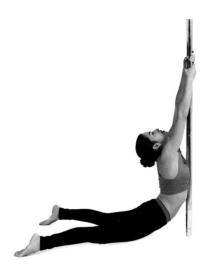

BACK EXTENSION

Face the pole with an upright posture and grasp it with both hands at chest level. Extend the arms while sliding toward the ground until the legs and pelvis make contact with the ground. Arch the back.

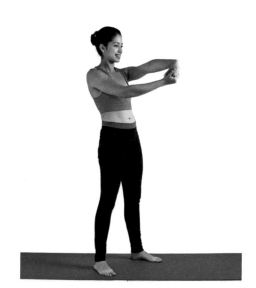

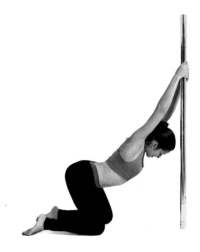

FINGER FLEXION AND EXTENSION

Stand in an upright position with the feet apart and the hips centralized. Extend both arms forward. Hold the dorsum of the hand and flex downward. Afterwards, pull the palmar side of the fingers, extending the wrist upward. Repeat with the opposite hand.

BACK AND SHOULDERS EXTENSION (A)

Assume a quadruped position. Facing the pole, grip it with both hands at shoulder level. Extend the arms while shifting the hips backward and extending the trunk upward. Arch the back.

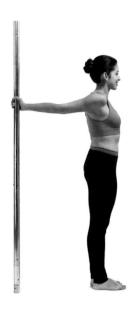

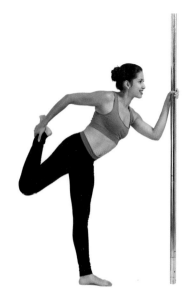

SHOULDER STRETCH (A)

Keeping the hips centralized and standing sideways to the pole, grasp the pole. Keep the arm extension parallel to the ground and turn the body to face away from the pole.

HIP FLEXORS STRETCH (A)

Maintaining an upright posture, face the pole, hold it by one hand at chest level, and hold the ankle by the opposite hand to slightly pull toward the glute.

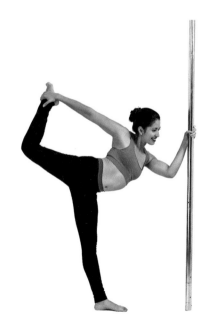

HIP FLEXORS
AND HAMSTRING STRETCH

Maintaining an upright posture, face the pole, hold it by one hand at chest level, and hold the ankle by the opposite hand to raise the leg backward. Lean the trunk forward while elevating the leg.

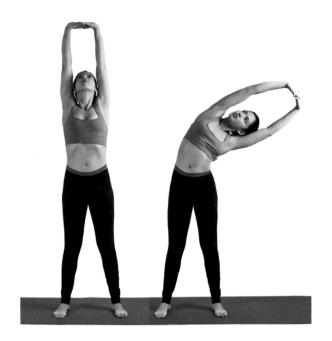

BACK LATERAL FLEXION

Stand in an upright position with the feet apart and the hips centralized. Interlock the fingers and raise them overhead to stretch. Bend the torso sideways. Opposite arm should be fully extended overhead. Repeat on the opposite side.

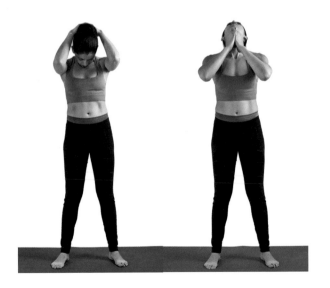

ROTATIONAL STRETCH

Stand in an upright position with the feet and the hips centralized. Flex the neck forward, backward, and sideways while applying mild pressure.

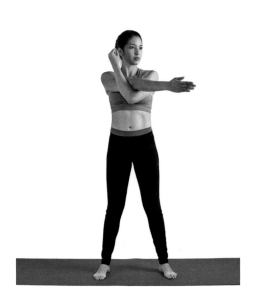

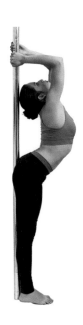

CROSS ARM STRETCH

Stand in an upright position with the feet apart and the hips centralized. Horizontally adduct one arm and use the opposite elbow to push it toward the chest.

BACK AND SHOULDERS EXTENSION (B)

Support the back on the pole and raise the arms overhead to grasp it. Push the trunk forward, keeping the back arched and the neck and arms extended.

BACK AND SHOULDERS EXTENSION (C)

With an upright posture and the toes touching the pole, face the pole. Grasp it at shoulder level and lean the hips backward while fully extending the arms.

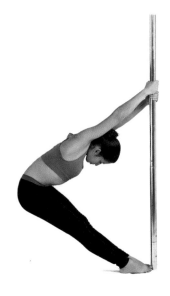

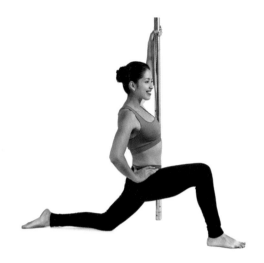

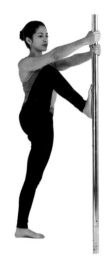

HIP FLEXORS STRETCH (B)

Adopt a lunge position facing sideways to the pole and grasp it with the near hand. Keep the back knee fully extended. Gently press the hips forward while slightly leaning the trunk backward. Repeat on the opposite side.

CALF STRETCH

Face the pole with an upright posture. Hold the pole by one hand at chest level. Support one foot on the pole above knee level with the knee flexed. Push the body against the pole to stretch the calves. Repeat on the opposite side.

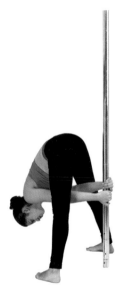

HAMSTRING STRETCH (BACK TO POLE)

Assume a standing position, supporting the back on the pole. Lean forward and hold the pole between the thighs. Bend the trunk forward and fully extend the elbows.

HIP FLEXORS STRETCH (C)

Adopt a lunge position, facing sideways to the pole, and hold it with the near hand. Keep the back knee supported on the ground and hold the ankle with the opposite hand, gently pulling the heel toward the glutes. Press the hips forward while slightly leaning the trunk backward. Repeat on the opposite side.

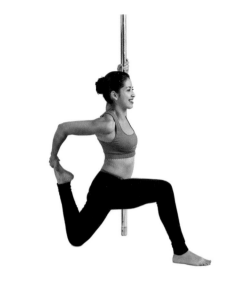

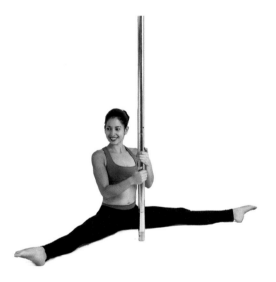

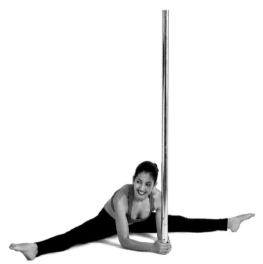

ADDUCTORS STRETCH

Sitting comfortably on the ground, hold the pole at chest level. Abduct and extend the legs sideways. Keep the back extended and gently lean forward.

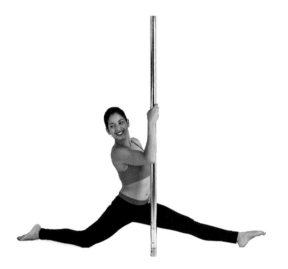

SPLIT

Adopt a lunge position, facing sideways to the pole, and hold it with the near hand. Keep the back knee fully extended. Gently press the hips forward while slightly leaning the trunk backward. When confident, extend the front leg and gradually slide forward.

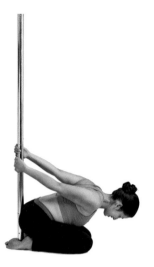

SHOULDER STRETCH (B)

Kneel with the tailbone in contact with the pole and extend the arms backward to hold the pole. Flex the neck and pull the body away to fully stretch the arms.

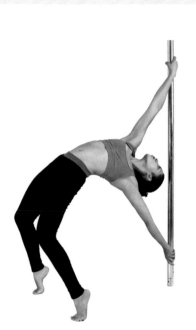

BACKBEND STRETCH

Assume a position sideways to the pole, holding with the near hand using a basic grip. Extend the far arm and hold the pole at a lower level while walking forward and arching the back.

BACK AND SHOULDERS EXTENSION (D)

Raise the arms overhead to hold the pole. Bend the trunk forward, keeping the back arched and supporting the chest on the pole. Extend the neck and arms upward.

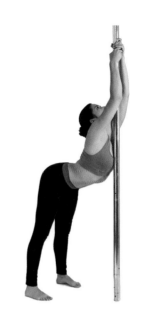

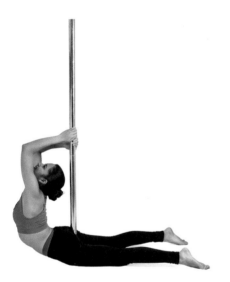

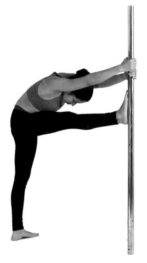

DEEP BACKBEND STRETCH

Assume a prone position with the pole between the thighs. Place the palms on the ground to raise and extend the upper back. When confident, extend the arms over the head to hold the pole. Keep the back arched.

HAMSTRING STRETCH

Face the pole with an upright posture. Hold the pole with one hand at chest level. Support one foot on the pole with knee flexion. Push against the pole so that the elbows and knee fully extend parallel to the ground. Repeat on the opposite side.

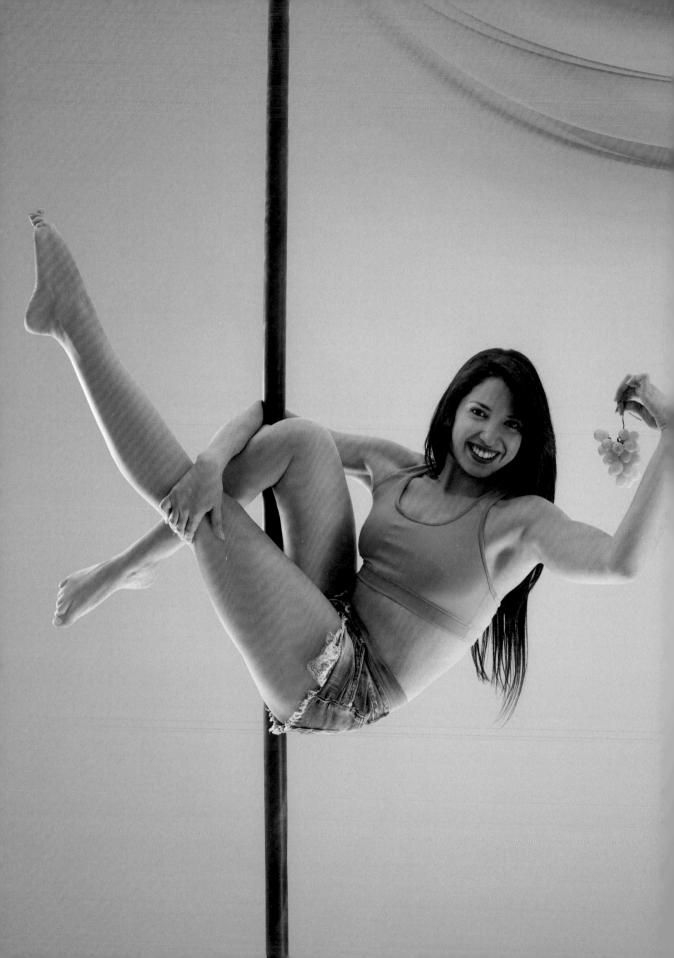

CHAPTER 12
WORKOUT NUTRITION PLAN

CHAPTER 12
WORKOUT NUTRITION PLAN

Dr. Cherryhan Salvedia is a clinical nutritionist who graduated from the National Nutrition Institute of Egypt. A registered physician, medical human physiologist, and basic life support instructor at the American Heart Association, Dr. Salvedia earned her M.B.Ch.B and M.D. at the Medical School of Cairo University and completed her internship program at Cairo University hospitals. She provides nutrition counseling for different age groups, helps obese children and adults with different medical disorders improve their quality of living, and develops nutrition plans for diabetic patients hand-in-hand with endocrinologists. She initiated nutrition education programs for the public and exercise trainers to encourage healthy lifestyles within her community, developed nutrition programs with Swedish psychologists and Egyptian psychiatrists for improving mental health in children with ADHD and autism, and created behavioral therapies for eating disorders. Dr. Salvedia also worked with certified Pilates instructors in Egypt to emphasize the need for strengthening core muscles and exercising in addition to proper nutrition. She embraces holistic nutrition plans and is constantly looking for innovation in support of leading a better life.

PRE-WORKOUT NUTRITION PLAN

Four hours before any exercise, nutrition should include complex carbohydrate meals of low glycemic index. Although fat is considered an alternative source of energy, meals should be lower in fat content. It is also important to hydrate well during this period to avoid dehydration during exercise.

These pre-workout meals should include complex carbohydrates. The maximum rate of absorption for carbohydrates is nearly 37 grams per hour in males and 27 grams per hour in females during the pre-workout period.

Two hours before exercising, we recommend liquid or semisolid meals that are lower in calories and that are made up of 30 grams of complex carbohydrates.

One hour before exercise, meals should be made up of liquids with a carbohydrate content of 30 grams.

POST-WORKOUT NUTRITION PLAN

This period of time is considered a window of opportunity. Glycogen stores in the liver and muscles need to be replenished at a rate of 40 grams per hour. Meals during this time should include carbohydrates and proteins at an average ratio of 4:1, depending on workout intensity level. Fats do not affect benefits of recovery, and instead slow it down.

In the first 15 minutes after exercise, up to 150% of lost fluids should be replaced.

Within two hours after exercise, meals should be high in glycemic index. It is also important to include meals which are rich in magnesium, manganese, and vitamin B6 to optimize the metabolic processes that are needed in glycogen synthesis and replenishment during this time.

PRE-WORKOUT MEALS

PASTA WITH SHRIMP

Preparation: 40 minutes   **Cooking:** 40 minutes   **Servings:** 1

INGREDIENTS

- ½ cup pasta
- 3 ounces shrimp
- 1 ounce spring onions
- ½ cup buttermilk
- 1 tablespoon corn starch
- 2 tablespoons fresh cilantro

- ½ teaspoon oregano
- 1 garlic clove, minced
- ¼ teaspoon garlic powder
- ¼ teaspoon salt
- ½ teaspoon black pepper

PREPARATION

1. In a saucepan, add a dash of salt to water and bring to boil. Add pasta.

2. In a skillet, allow oil to heat, then add the spring onions and minced garlic for 1 minute over medium heat.

3. Add the shrimp, oregano, cilantro, salt, and pepper and sauté until shrimp is cooked through.

4. Lower the heat and add the cooked pasta.

5. In a separate pan, bring buttermilk to a simmer, then whisk in the corn starch until the milk thickens.

6. Add the thickened buttermilk to the pasta and continue to heat for another 3 to 5 minutes.

NUTRITIONAL INFORMATION

- Calories: 421
- Carbohydrates: 64 grams

- Protein: 30 grams
- Fat: 5 grams

Oregano is a medicinal herb that has been used in cooking for thousands of years. It has very high levels of antioxidants and vitamin K. Vitamin K is important for maintaining bone density and blood clotting. It is also a good source of iron, calcium, magnesium, vitamin E, omega fatty acids, manganese, and tryptophan.

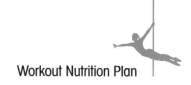

SUSHI ROLLS

Preparation: 30 minutes   **Cooking:** 30 minutes   **Servings:** 1

INGREDIENTS

- Nori paper
- ½ cup short grain rice (preferably glutinous rice)
- 1 cup water
- ¼ cup sushi vinegar

- 1 ounce crab meat, salmon, or tuna
- 1 tablespoon cream cheese
- ¼ avocado
- 1 tablespoon lemon juice

PREPARATION

1. Slice avocado lengthwise and sprinkle with lemon juice.

2. In a saucepan, add rice to one cup of water and cook over low heat until soft.

3. Add sushi vinegar to warm rice and allow to cool slightly.

4. Wrap the rolling mat with a plastic wrap and spread out the Nori sheet with the smooth surface down.

5. Starting in the center, gently spread the sushi rice toward the edges.

6. Place the crab meat, salmon, or tuna along the near edge.

7. Place the avocado slices and cheese next to the seafood toward the front edge, then roll with the help of the rolling mat.

8. Cut off the edges and slice the sushi roll into 6 pieces.

NUTRITIONAL INFORMATION

- Calories: 621
- Carbohydrates: 111.5 grams

- Protein: 14.5 grams
- Fat: 13 grams

Crab meat is rich in selenium. It contains 12 times the amount of selenium found in beef. It also contains nearly 56 times the amount found in salmon, chicken, and beef. Copper is involved in the absorption, storage, and metabolism of iron, thus it is important in the formation of red blood cells. One hundred grams of crab provides 62% of the daily recommended copper values for adults.

ADOBO CHICKEN AND BOK CHOY

Preparation: 10 minutes   **Cooking:** 30 minutes   **Servings:** 1

INGREDIENTS

- 3 ounces chicken breast, cubed
- ½ small onion
- 1 garlic clove, minced
- ½ tablespoon dark soy sauce
- 1 tablespoon vinegar
- 1 teaspoon honey
- 1 tablespoon olive oil
- 1 bay leaf
- 1 teaspoon sea salt
- Dash of black pepper
- 3 leaves of bok choy

PREPARATION

1. Mix dark soy sauce and vinegar in a small bowl to form a marinade, then add honey, salt, and pepper.

2. Sauté onion and garlic over medium heat for 2 minutes, then add chicken and stir for another 3 minutes.

3. Add bay leaf and marinade.

4. Lower the heat, then simmer for 20 minutes until tender.

5. Serve with bok choy.

NUTRITIONAL INFORMATION

- Calories: 318
- Carbohydrates: 18 grams
- Protein: 21 grams
- Fat: 18 grams

Bok choy is a powerhouse of vitamin C, which improves cardiovascular health, and vitamin E, which helps maximize the health benefits of the meal as both vitamins work synergistically. It is rich in vitamin K, and calcium is highly bioavailable.

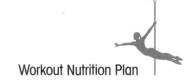

GRILLED CHICKEN TACOS

Preparation: 30 minutes   **Cooking:** 15 minutes   **Servings:** 1

INGREDIENTS

- 3 ounce chicken breast
- 1 small cucumber, julienned
- 1 small red pepper, julienned
- 1 small yellow pepper, julienned

- 2 medium flour tortillas (7-8")*
- 1 tablespoon olive oil
- ½ teaspoon salt
- ½ teaspoon black pepper

*For a gluten-free recipe, use corn tortillas instead of flour.

PREPARATION

1. Mix olive oil with salt and pepper and coat the chicken breast.

2. Broil on each side until firm, then shred.

3. Mix the vegetables with the shredded chicken.

4. Divide the mix into to the tortillas.

5. Fold the tortillas in half and grill for 2 minutes before serving.

NUTRITIONAL INFORMATION

- Calories: 568
- Carbohydrates: 57 grams

- Protein: 28 grams
- Fat: 25.3 grams

Bell peppers contain over 30 different types of carotenoids. To maximize vitamin C and carotenoid content, allow peppers to ripen before consumption. As overheating destroys phytonutrient content—specifically Luteolin flavonoid—it is preferable to ingest them ripe and raw.

TUNA FISH CAKES AND GREEN BEANS WITH POMEGRANATE SEEDS

Preparation: 20 minutes   **Cooking:** 30 minutes   **Servings:** 1

INGREDIENTS

For the tuna fish cake:

- 2 ounces tuna
- 2 tablespoon whisked egg
- 1 tablespoon lemon juice
- 1 tablespoon olive oil
- 1 tablespoon white onion, diced

- 1 tablespoon mozzarella
- 1 tablespoon bread crumbs
- 1 teaspoon salt
- 1 teaspoon black pepper

For the green beans with pomegranate seeds:

- ½ cup (75 grams) green beans
- ¼ cup (22 grams) pomegranate seeds
- 1 tablespoon balsamic vinegar
- 2 teaspoon olive oil

- 1 teaspoon minced garlic
- ¼ teaspoon salt
- ¼ teaspoon black pepper

PREPARATION

For the tuna fish cake:

1. Fold together tuna and diced onions.

2. Combine eggs, lemon juice, mozzarella, bread crumbs, salt, and pepper to form a paste.

3. Add paste to tuna mixture, then shape into three thick patties.

4. Place tuna patties in a pan brushed with olive oil.

5. Bake at 320 ˚F for 5 minutes per side.

For the green beans and pomegranate seeds:

1. Heat olive oil in a skillet and add minced garlic. Sauté for 1 minute.

2. Add salt and pepper, then stir fry green beans for 5 minutes.

3. Add balsamic vinegar and stir for another minute.

4. Serve green beans with pomegranate seeds sprinkled on the top.

NUTRITIONAL INFORMATION

- Calories: 577
- Carbohydrates: 29 grams
- Protein: 23
- Fat: 41

Green beans are very rich in fiber, making them good for digestion. They are also good sources of vitamin C and folic acid, as well as calcium, silicon, iron, manganese, potassium, and copper. Green beans also contain phytates and lectins (though at lower levels than other members of the bean family). Phytates bind and prevent absorption of calcium and zinc, while lectins bind proteins that affect digestion. Cooking can reduce these levels, but it is not recommended to ingest green beans if you have mineral deficiencies.

WORCESTERSHIRE STEAK AND LEMON-GINGER ASPARAGUS

Preparation: 20 minutes   **Cooking:** 50 minutes   **Servings:** 1

INGREDIENTS

For the Worcestershire steak:

- 3 ounce steak
- 2 tablespoon balsamic vinegar
- 2 tablespoon Worcestershire sauce
- 2 tablespoon low-sodium soy sauce

- 1 tablespoon olive oil
- 1 teaspoon Dijon mustard
- 1 teaspoon minced garlic
- Dash of salt and pepper

For the lemon-ginger asparagus:

- 120 grams asparagus
- 1 tablespoon olive oil
- 1 tablespoon red wine vinegar
- 1 teaspoon Dijon mustard

- 1 teaspoon grated ginger
- 1 garlic clove, minced
- Zest of one lemon
- ¼ teaspoon salt

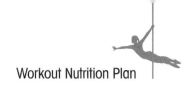

PREPARATION

For the Worcestershire steak:

1. Combine oil, vinegar, Worcestershire sauce, low-sodium soy sauce, Dijon mustard, garlic, salt, and pepper.

2. Marinate the steak.

3. Grill or broil to taste.

For the lemon-ginger asparagus:

1. Preheat oven at 400 ˚F.

2. Combine olive oil, vinegar, Dijon mustard, garlic, ginger, lemon zest, and salt.

3. Trim ends of asparagus and fold into the sauce.

4. Spread asparagus in a single layer on a baking sheet and bake for 8 minutes on each side. Serve warm.

NUTRITIONAL INFORMATION

- Calories: 508
- Carbohydrates: 25 grams
- Protein: 21 grams
- Fat: 36 grams

Lemon peel helps eradicate toxic elements in the body. They contain more vitamins than lemon juice, including vitamin C, vitamin A, beta-carotene, folate, calcium, magnesium, and potassium.

Asparagus is rich in fiber and vitamin B complex. It is also an excellent source of vitamin K, folate, copper, selenium, vitamin C, and vitamin E. It is a very good source of zinc and iron. The recommended blanching time for asparagus is 3-5 minutes depending on thickness to maintain these levels of micronutrients.

CREAMY CHICKEN WITH HOT BISCUITS

Preparation: 45 minutes   **Cooking:** 45 minutes   **Servings:** 1

INGREDIENTS

For the creamy chicken:

- 3 ounce chicken breast, cubed
- ½ cup frozen green peas
- 1 cup low-sodium chicken broth*
- 3 tablespoon heavy cream
- 1 tablespoon corn starch

- 1 tablespoon butter
- ¼ teaspoon garlic powder
- ¼ teaspoon salt
- ½ teaspoon black pepper
- ¼ cup sliced almonds

For the hot biscuits:

- ¼ cup flour
- ¼ cup buttermilk
- 1 tablespoon butter

- ¼ tablespoon baking powder
- ¼ teaspoon salt
- Dash of baking soda

*Replace the low-sodium chicken broth with a sodium-free chicken broth or water to reduce the salt content of the meal.

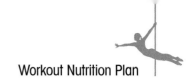

PREPARATION

For the creamy chicken:

1. Melt butter in a large skillet, then add chicken, peas, garlic, salt, and pepper

2. Stir over medium heat until chicken and peas are cooked then lower the heat.

3. In a separate saucepan, simmer heavy cream and chicken broth, then whisk in corn starch until the mixture thickens.

4. Add cream to chicken and cook for another 5 minutes.

5. Serve chicken with almond slices sprinkled on top.

For the hot biscuits:

1. Preheat the oven to 450 ˚F then combine flour, baking soda, baking powder, and salt in a large bowl.

2. Mix butter into the dry ingredients until it resembles a coarse meal.

3. Add buttermilk, and mix gently until combined into a very wet dough (add more buttermilk if needed).

4. Gently pat the dough out to half-inch thickness and gently fold it several times, then press it gently out to half an inch thick again.

5. Cut out biscuits using a cookie cutter.

6. Place the biscuits close to each other on a baking sheet to get them to rise higher and have softer edges.

7. Bake for 12 minutes. Do not overbake!

NUTRITIONAL INFORMATION

- Calories: 744
- Carbohydrates: 61 grams
- Protein: 35 grams
- Fat: 40 grams

Green peas are rich in dietary fiber. Like many other green foods, they are good sources of vitamin K, folic acid, manganese, magnesium, copper, iron, potassium, and molybdenum. They also provide choline.

HONEY-GARLIC CHICKEN THIGHS

Preparation: 10 minutes   **Cooking:** 60 minutes   **Servings:** 1

INGREDIENTS

- 2 chicken thighs
- ¼ cup water
- 1 tablespoon low-sodium soy sauce
- 1 tablespoon ketchup
- 1 tablespoon honey
- ½ teaspoon dried basil
- 1 garlic clove, minced

PREPARATION

1. Mix all ingredients to form a marinade for the chicken. Marinate chicken for 30 minutes.

2. Bake the chicken thighs at 325 °F for 40 minutes.

Serve with ½ cup steamed rice.

NUTRITIONAL INFORMATION

- Calories: 624
- Carbohydrates: 98 grams
- Protein: 37 grams
- Fat: 8 grams

Boneless chicken thighs of the same amount provide more calories but are higher in protein.

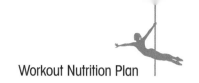

THAI CASHEWS WITH CHICKEN

Preparation: 15 minutes   **Cooking:** 30 minutes   **Servings:** 1

INGREDIENTS

For the chicken:

- 3 ounces chicken breast, sliced
- 1 garlic clove, minced
- 1 medium red chili, seeded and diced

- 1 tablespoon vegetable oil
- 1 small yellow onion, sliced
- ¼ cups raw cashew nuts

For the sauce:

- 1 teaspoon low-sodium soy sauce
- 1 tablespoon sweet dark soy sauce
- 1 tablespoon fish sauce

- 1 tablespoon brown sugar
- 1 tablespoon water

PREPARATION

1. Combine all the sauce ingredients in a small bowl and set aside.
2. In a small wok, heat the oil over medium heat.
3. Sauté cashews until they turn brown, then set aside.
4. Stir fry the garlic, onion, and red chili for 3 minutes.
5. Add the sliced chicken and stir fry until chicken turns opaque and is cooked through.
6. Add the cashews and stir fry for another minute, then add the sauce to the wok.
7. Lower the heat and continue to stir fry for 3 minutes.
8. Serve immediately.

NUTRITIONAL INFORMATION

- Calories: 625
- Carbohydrates: 46 grams

- Protein: 30 grams
- Fat: 35.6 grams

Red chili peppers are rich in vitamin C which represents about 239% of a 2,000-calorie diet. Fish sauce is also rich in magnesium which represents about 43% of a 2,000-calorie diet.

BAKED POTATOES WITH PESTO

Preparation: 10 minutes   **Cooking:** 25 minutes   **Servings:** 1

INGREDIENTS

- For the baked potatoes:
- 250 g small white potatoes
- 1 tablespoon vegetable oil

For the pesto:

- ½ cup fresh basil
- 1 tablespoon water
- 1 tablespoon olive oil
- 1 tablespoon nutritional yeast

- 1 tablespoon walnuts
- 1 garlic clove, minced
- Dash of salt

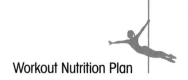

PREPARATION

For the potatoes:

1. Bring a pot of salted water to a boil.

2. Cut potatoes in half and boil for about 15 minutes or until tender.

3. Preheat oven to 320 ˚F and spread potatoes on a baking sheet.

4. Slightly flatten the potatoes and bake for 5 minutes.

5. Drizzle pesto on top for serving.

For the pesto:

1. Combine all ingredients in a food processor until smooth paste is formed.

2. Add water if needed for thinner consistency.

3. Pesto can be kept in the refrigerator for several days.

NUTRITIONAL INFORMATION

- Calories: 572
- Carbohydrates: 50 grams
- Protein: 12 grams
- Fat: 36 grams

There are 35 different types of basils! Holy basil (known as tulsi in India) has the most healing and anti-inflammatory properties. Basil contains at least six types of essential oils and is a powerful adaptogen. It fights stress, depression, and diseases.

CHICKEN MUSHROOM SOUP AND CORNBREAD

Preparation: 30 minutes   **Cooking:** 45 minutes

INGREDIENTS

For the chicken mushroom soup (1 serving):

- 3 ounce chicken breast, diced
- ½ medium carrots, diced
- ½ celery stalk, diced
- 2 ounces fresh mushrooms, sliced
- 1 garlic clove, minced
- 1 tablespoon diced green onion
- 2 tablespoon sour cream

- 1 tablespoon butter
- ½ tablespoon olive oil
- 1 tablespoon flour
- 1 cup water or no-sodium chicken broth
- ¼ teaspoon dried thyme
- ¼ teaspoon salt
- ¼ teaspoon black pepper

For the cornbread (16 servings):

- 1 cup yellow cornmeal
- 1 egg
- 1 tablespoon sugar
- 1 tablespoon baking powder

- ¼ teaspoon salt
- 120 g creamed corn
- ½ cup sour cream
- ½ cup vegetable oil

PREPARATION

For the chicken mushroom soup:

1. In a large saucepan over medium heat, heat oil and butter, then add chicken, carrot, and celery.

2. Stir until chicken is cooked, then add mushrooms and continue stirring.

3. In a separate pan, allow chicken broth to simmer, then whisk in sour cream.

4. Add flour, thyme, salt, and pepper, and continue stirring.

5. Add cream mixture to chicken and lower the heat.

6. Cover the saucepan and leave to simmer for 15 minutes.

Corn bread (16 servings)

1. Preheat oven to 420°F with a 10-inch skillet inside.

2. In a bowl, combine cornmeal, baking powder, salt, and sugar.

3. In another bowl, whisk together egg, creamed corn, sour cream, and oil.

4. Add the egg mixture to the cornmeal mixture and stir to form a batter.

5. Rub the skillet with 1 tablespoon oil and pour the batter in.

6. Bake for 20 minutes, then cut into 16 pieces and serve hot.

NUTRITIONAL INFORMATION

Soup

- Calories: 421
- Carbohydrates: 25 grams
- Protein: 24 grams
- Fat: 25 grams

One serving of corn bread

- Calories: 128
- Carbohydrates: 10.3 grams
- Protein: 1.4 grams
- Fat: 9 grams

For a gluten-free meal, replace flour with corn flour in the soup. If you are looking to lose weight, replace the cornbread with two toasted slices of bread.

Dried thyme is another herb that is rich in Iron. It is also a good source of calcium, magnesium, and vitamin C.

LENTIL SOUP

Preparation: 15 minutes   **Cooking:** 30 minutes   **Servings:** 1

INGREDIENTS

- ½ cup of water
- ¼ cup (50 g) lentils
- 1 medium carrot, chopped
- 1 garlic clove, minced
- 1 tablespoon sliced yellow onions
- ¼ teaspoon dried coriander
- Dash of salt and pepper

PREPARATION

1. Heat the oil over medium heat, then add garlic and onions.

2. Add water, lentils, carrots, coriander, salt, and pepper, then allow to boil for 30 minutes or until the carrots are tender.

3. Blend the soup in a food processor until smooth.

4. Serve with two toasted bread slices.

NUTRITIONAL INFORMATION

- Calories: 209
- Carbohydrates: 38 grams
- Protein: 13 grams
- Fat: 0.5 grams

This is a very healthy vegetarian meal—26% of its calories are from protein and it has no fat. It is rich in soluble fibers, reducing cholesterol levels and insoluble fiber content to maintain a healthy functioning gut. It is also a good source of magnesium and folate. Magnesium improves blood flow, while folate lowers homocysteine levels (a risk factor for heart disease). It is also a good source of iron.

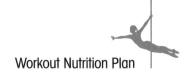

SWEET POTATO AND CARROT GINGER-CURRY SOUP

Preparation: 10 minutes   **Cooking:** 40 minutes   **Servings:** 1

INGREDIENTS

- ½ small shallot, chopped
- 2 medium carrots, cubed
- 1 large sweet potato, cubed
- 1 cup water

- 1 tablespoon oil
- 2 teaspoon grated ginger
- 1 teaspoon curry powder
- Dash of salt

PREPARATION

1. In a saucepan, heat oil over medium heat, then add shallots, sweet potatoes, and carrots.
2. Add water, grated ginger, curry powder, and salt, then lower the heat.
3. Cover the pan and allow vegetables to simmer for 30 minutes or until tender.
4. Blend the vegetables and liquid in a food processor until smooth.

NUTRITIONAL INFORMATION

- Calories: 461
- Carbohydrates: 70 grams

- Protein: 7 grams
- Fat: 17 grams

Curry powder is made up of a large number of ingredients which vary from one region to another, but the most common ingredients include turmeric, coriander, cardamom, and sweet basil. Coriander boosts the immune system and guards against intestinal infections. Cardamom and sweet basil are natural vasodilators which improve blood flow and heart health. Some curry powders contain ginger, so check its ingredients before adding additional ginger to this recipe. Curry powder is a potential irritant to the gall bladder and has blood-thinning properties, so it is recommended to consult a physician before use.

BAKED SPRING EGGS AND BEANS

Preparation: 40 minutes   **Cooking:** 90 minutes   **Servings:** 1

INGREDIENTS

For the baked spring egg:

- 1 egg
- 1 tablespoon diced red bell pepper
- 1 tablespoon diced green bell pepper

- 1 tablespoon diced red onions
- Dash of salt and black pepper

For the beans:

- ¼ cup dried white beans
- 1 garlic clove, minced
- 1 medium tomato, blended

- 1 small onion, grated
- 1 tablespoon vegetable oil
- Dash of salt and pepper

PREPARATION

For the baked spring egg:

1. Grease a cupcake pan or other very small pan with oil.

2. Combine diced vegetables with the egg.

3. Pour into the pan.

4. Bake at 320 ˚F for 10 minutes.

For the beans:

1. Soak the dried white beans in water for 30 minutes or until swollen.

2. Over medium heat, bring the beans to a boil, then lower the heat and simmer for about 20 minutes.

3. Allow the beans to cool then drain, meanwhile, grate the onions and blend the tomato

4. Sauté the onion and garlic with vegetable oil, then add the blended tomato and keep stirring for 3 minutes.

5. Add the white beans, stir, and then cover. Simmer for 10 minutes.

6. Serve with baked spring egg.

NUTRITIONAL INFORMATION

- Calories: 449
- Carbohydrates: 40.3 grams
- Protein: 21 grams
- Fat: 22.6 grams

White beans are loaded with antioxidants and provide a good supply of detoxifying molybdenum. They are rich in vitamin B1, needed for brain function, and folate, which reduces homocysteine levels, thus improving heart health. Like other beans, they are low in glycemic levels, and they are rich in fiber, both soluble and insoluble. Soluble fiber helps reduce cholesterol levels and insoluble fiber improves digestive health. White beans have vast quantities of magnesium which **maintains the electrical potential across muscle membranes** and **helps handle stress**. It is also necessary for bone health.

BLACK BEANS, EGG, AND HASHBROWNS

Preparation: 30 minutes   **Cooking:** 40 minutes   **Servings:** 1

INGREDIENTS

For the black beans and egg:

- 2 ounce canned black beans, drained and rinsed
- 1 tablespoon salsa
- 1 teaspoon oil

For the hashbrowns:

- 1 medium potato, grated
- 1 teaspoon flour

- ¼ sliced avocado (optional)
- Dash of salt and pepper
- 1 egg

- 2 teaspoon whisked egg

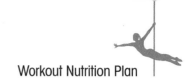

PREPARATION

For the black beans and egg:

1. In a small pan, heat the black beans with oil and salsa for 3 minutes.

2. Scramble the egg and serve it with the black beans and avocado slices (optional).

For the hashbrowns:

1. Combine grated potato, egg, and flour.

2. Divide into two patties.

3. Grill in a non-stick pan for 10 minutes per side.

NUTRITIONAL INFORMATION

- Calories: 531

- Carbohydrates: 65 grams

- Protein: 25 grams

- Fat: 19 grams

Black beans have strong antioxidant properties attributed mostly to their high concentrations of **anthocyanins** such as delphinidin, petunidin, and malvidin. Like other beans, they have lectin which is toxic, so they should be well cooked before eating. Black beans are also rich in glutamine, magnesium, iron, and potassium. They have a low glycemic index level and can therefore aid in weight loss.

PRE-WORKOUT SNACKS

RICE PAPER ROLLS

Preparation: 20 minutes   **Servings:** 1

INGREDIENTS

For the rice paper rolls:

- 2 rice papers (8")
- ¼ apple, sliced
- ½ mango, sliced
- 3 small yellow plums, sliced

For the peanut-butter dipping sauce:

- 1½ tablespoon peanut butter
- 1 tablespoon white vinegar
- 1 garlic clove, minced
- 2 tablespoon milk
- ½ teaspoon chili powder (optional)

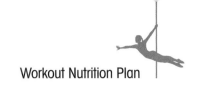

PREPARATION

For the rice paper rolls:

1. Fill a large bowl with warm water and submerge the rice papers.

2. Spread out the dampened rice papers with the smooth surface down.

3. Place mango slices at the lower part of the rice paper, apple slices in the middle, and the plum slices at the top of the paper, and fold right and left edges in.

4. Start rolling the papers from bottom to top. Firmly hold all slices and rice paper as you roll, and it will seal itself.

For the peanut-butter dipping sauce:

1. Mix all ingredients together and warm for 30 seconds in the microwave until smooth.

2. Adjust thickness with water or milk, according to your taste.

NUTRITIONAL INFORMATION

- Calories: 333
- Carbohydrates: 44 grams
- Protein: 10 grams
- Fat: 13 grams

Plums are good sources of dietary fiber as well as sorbitol and isatin. They encourage secretion in the bowel, which benefits gut health and is effective in treating digestive disorders like constipations. Plums have impressive quantities of bioactive compounds including phenols, flavonoids, phytonutrients, and vitamin C, rendering them high in antioxidants and anti-inflammatory properties.

SWEET POTATO WEDGES AND MAPLE-FIG SAUCE

Preparation: 20 minutes   **Cooking:** 15 minutes   **Servings:** 1

INGREDIENTS

For the sweet potato wedges:

- 1 medium sweet potato, peeled and sliced lengthwise
- ½ teaspoon sugar
- Dash of salt and black pepper
- Dash of red pepper

- For the maple-fig sauce
- 1 tablespoon fig jam
- 1 tablespoon sour cream
- ½ tablespoon mayonnaise
- 1 teaspoon maple syrup

PREPARATION

For the sweet potato wedges:

1. Preheat oven to 475 ˚F.

2. In a small bowl, mix sugar, salt, black pepper, and red pepper, and toss with sweet potato to coat.

3. Spread sweet potato on a baking sheet with cut sides down and bake for 10 minutes.

For the maple-fig sauce:

1. Mix all ingredients together.

2. Refrigerate until use.

NUTRITIONAL INFORMATION

- Calories: 359
- Carbohydrates: 53 grams

- Protein: 3 grams
- Fat: 15 grams

Figs are good sources of minerals, including magnesium, manganese, calcium, copper, and potassium, as well as vitamin K and vitamin B6. Their nutritional values increase when dried. They are also rich in dietary fiber and therefore regulate blood sugar and help in weight management. However, they also contain fructose, so it is recommended that they be consumed in moderation.

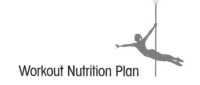

BANANA BREAD

Preparation: 15 minutes   **Cooking:** 60 minutes   **Servings:** 12

INGREDIENTS

- 2 cups plain flour
- 2 cups mashed bananas
- 2 eggs
- ½ cup brown sugar
- ½ cup butter
- 1 teaspoon baking soda
- ¼ teaspoon salt

PREPARATION

1. Preheat the oven to 360°F and grease a loaf pan.

2. In a large bowl, combine flour, baking soda, and salt. In another bowl, combine sugar and butter, then add mashed bananas and beaten eggs.

3. Add the banana mixture to the flour mixture and stir to blend, then pour batter into the loaf pan.

4. Bake for 60 minutes.

5. Allow bread to cool, then serve.

NUTRITIONAL INFORMATION

Each serving (30 grams)

- Calories: 250
- Carbohydrates: 36 grams
- Protein: 4 grams
- Fat: 10 grams

Bananas are rich in potassium which maintains fluid levels in the body and regulates the movement of nutrients and waste products in and out of the cells. It helps muscles and the heart contract properly and allows nerves to respond normally. It can also reduce the effects of sodium on blood pressure in hypertensive people. Healthy kidneys are needed to maintain normal potassium blood concentration, thus bananas, along with other potassium-rich foods, should be consumed in moderation.

BLUEBERRY OATMEAL BARS

Preparation: 30 minutes   **Cooking:** 40 minutes   **Servings:** 12

INGREDIENTS

For the filling:

- 1 cup blueberries
- 1 ½ tablespoon chia seeds

For the bars:

- 1 cup oat or wheat flour
- 1 cup classic oats
- 2 tablespoon brown sugar
- ½ teaspoon baking soda
- ½ teaspoon cinnamon

- 1 tablespoon maple syrup

- ¼ teaspoon salt
- ½ cup unsweetened apple sauce
- ¼ cup maple syrup
- ¼ cup coconut oil

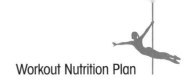

PREPARATION

1. Stir blueberries, maple syrup, and chia seeds over medium heat for 15 minutes.

2. Smash the blueberries and set the filling aside.

3. Combine the oat flour, classic oats, brown sugar, baking soda, cinnamon, and salt in a large bowl.

4. Stir in the unsweetened apple sauce, maple syrup, and coconut oil.

5. Preheat the oven at 325 ° F and grease an 8 x 8 baking pan.

6. Spread half of the oat mixture onto the baking pan, then spread the blueberry chia jam on top of the oat mixture. Top with the remaining oat mixture.

7. Bake for 40 minutes, then allow to cool before cutting into 12 bars.

8. Store in the refrigerator.

9. Recommendation: Post-workout snack bar can be eaten with a half cup of skim milk.

NUTRITIONAL INFORMATION

Each serving (60 grams)

- Calories: 106
- Carbohydrates: 12 grams
- Protein: 1 gram
- Fat: 6 grams

Oats are rich in a specific type of fiber called beta-glucan. This particular type of fiber is known to help lower cholesterol levels. One cup (81 g) of dry oats contains 8.2 g of fiber which is about one-third of the daily requirement for fiber. Oats are gluten free, but if grown in the same fields as wheat or barley, they are sometimes contaminated by glutenave from these crops.

MASHED SWEET POTATO AND MAPLE SYRUP

Preparation: 10 minutes   **Cooking:** 40 minutes   **Servings:** 1

INGREDIENTS

- 1 medium sweet potato
- 1 tablespoon maple syrup
- 1/8 cup pecans
- Dash of nutmeg
- Dash of cinnamon
- Dash of ground cloves

PREPARATION

1. Place sweet potato on a baking sheet and bake at 420 °F for 30 minutes.

2. Over medium heat in a small skillet, melt the butter until its color changes to a golden brown and it smells nutty.

3. Peel and mash the sweet potato, then add nutmeg, cinnamon, and ground cloves.

4. Combine the maple syrup and butter, then add some to the mashed sweet potato.

5. Pour the rest over top of the mashed sweet potato and sprinkle with pecans.

NUTRITIONAL INFORMATION

- Calories: 302
- Carbohydrates: 47 grams
- Protein: 3.6 grams
- Fat: 11 grams

Maple syrup is a preferred choice over honey considering its lower calorie count. It is a good source of both zinc and magnesium, which play a key role in strengthening the immune system. Zinc also enhances the performance of the endothelial cells which line the blood vessels and protects endothelial cells against damage from excess cholesterol in the blood stream.

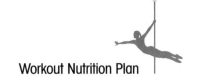

ALMOND-APRICOT SNACK BARS

Preparation: 30   **Cooking:** 10   **Servings:** 12

INGREDIENTS

- 1 cup dried apricots
- 1 cup unsweetened coconut flakes
- ½ cup pitted dates
- ½ cup whole almonds
- ½ cup almond flakes
- 2 tablespoon almond butter

PREPARATION

1. Combine apricots, dates, whole almonds, and almond butter in a food processor, then place in a bowl.

2. Preheat oven to 380 ˚F and toast coconut and almond flakes for 7 minutes.

3. Add toasted coconut and almond flakes to the apricot mixture and mix using your hands.

4. Line an 8.5 x 8.5 baking sheet with plastic wrap, then press the mixture into the pan using the palm of your hand.

5. Freeze for 15 minutes, then cut into 12 bars.

6. Bars may be stored in the refrigerator or freezer for up to 2 weeks.

NUTRITIONAL INFORMATION

- Calories: 150
- Carbohydrates: 14.3 grams
- Protein: 3 grams
- Fat: 9 grams

Dried fruit offers some benefits over fresh fruits as they boost energy, but they are higher in sugar content. Dried fruits—particularly figs, raisins, plums, and apricots—are rich sources of dietary fiber and iron. Apricots are a significant source of potassium which maintains proper fluid balance and helps in muscle function. Apricots contain significant amounts of both soluble and insoluble fiber. They are especially high in soluble fiber which helps maintain normal blood glucose and cholesterol levels.

VANILLA CHIA PUDDING

Preparation: 60 minutes   **Servings:** 1

INGREDIENTS

- ½ cup unsweetened almond milk
- 2 tablespoon chia seeds
- 1 teaspoon honey
- ¼ teaspoon vanilla extract
- Nuts, fruits, or coconut flakes for toppings (optional)

PREPARATION

1. Stir all ingredients together.

2. Place the mixture in an airtight container and refrigerate overnight.

3. Serve with any topping of your choice.

NUTRITIONAL INFORMATION

- Calories: 161
- Carbohydrates: 15 grams
- Protein: 5 grams
- Fat: 9 grams

Chia seeds can absorb 27 times their weight in water to form a thick gel; it is recommended to not give them to children and to mix chia seeds with liquids, especially for those with a history of swallowing problems. They provide more omega 3 fatty acids than flaxseeds, and they are good sources of phosphorous, calcium, and fiber.

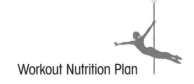

APRICOT-VANILLA CASHEW BARS

Preparation: 75 minutes   **Servings:** 12

INGREDIENTS

- 1 cup dried apricots
- I cup cashews
- ¼ cup pitted dates

- 1 tablespoon cashew butter
- ½ teaspoon vanilla extract

PREPARATION

1. Mix all ingredients in a blender or food processor (it will be sticky!).

2. Line an 8 x 8 baking sheet with parchment paper and flatten the mixture into the baking sheet using another piece of parchment paper.

3. Refrigerate for an hour.

4. Cut into 12 bars.

NUTRITIONAL INFORMATION

- Calories: 124
- Carbohydrates: 12 grams

- Protein: 4 grams
- Fat: 6.6 grams

Cashew butter is an excellent way to replace animal fat and proteins. It is rich in monosaturated and polyunsaturated fats which help in managing weight and reducing the build-up of fat and cholesterol in the heart. It is also rich in antioxidants such as lutein and zeaxanthin which play important roles in eye health.

CINNAMON SNACK BARS

Preparation: 30 minutes   **Servings:** 12

INGREDIENTS

- 1 cup unsalted cashews
- 1 cup soft pitted dates
- ½ cup rolled oats
- ½ cup protein powder

- 2 tablespoon nonfat milk
- ½ teaspoon cinnamon
- ¼ teaspoon salt

PREPARATION

1. Combine cashews and dates in a blender until a sticky ball is formed.

2. Add protein powder, rolled oats, cinnamon, and salt and process once more until oats are broken up.

3. Add nonfat milk and combine well.

4. Line an 8 x 8 baking sheet with plastic wrap and spread out the mixture.

5. Freeze for 15 minutes, then cut into 12 bars.

6. Bars may be stored in the refrigerator for up to a month.

NUTRITIONAL INFORMATION

- Calories: 153
- Carbohydrates: 12.5 grams

- Protein: 10 grams
- Fat: 7 grams

Cinnamon can be beneficial in pain management as it reduces swelling and inflammation. Some studies show that cinnamon helps to relieve muscles soreness and PMS pains. Cinnamon also speeds up metabolism as it takes a little extra energy to metabolize, thus allowing more calories to be burnt and aiding weight loss. Cinnamon is also rich in antioxidants, protecting cells from damage.

SWEET POTATO CASSEROLE

Preparation: 10 minutes   **Cooking:** 90 minutes   **Servings:** 4

INGREDIENTS

- 2 large sweet potatoes
- ½ cup nonfat milk
- ¼ cup flour
- 2 tablespoon white sugar
- 2 tablespoon brown sugar
- 1 tablespoon butter

PREPARATION

1. Bake sweet potatoes at 420 ˚F for 60 minutes.
2. Peel and mash the sweet potatoes.
3. Mix white sugar and milk, then add to the mashed sweet potatoes and mix.
4. Spread the mashed sweet potatoes in a baking dish.
5. In a separate bowl, cream together the butter and brown sugar.
6. Add the flour, then continue mixing using your hands.
7. Spread mixture on top of the mashed sweet potatoes.
8. Bake at 420 ˚F for 15 to 20 minutes.

NUTRITIONAL INFORMATION

- Calories: 220
- Carbohydrates: 43 grams
- Protein: 3 grams
- Fat: 4 grams

Sweet potatoes have different varieties including white, yellow, pink, and purple. They are considered one of the richest sources of vitamin A—a large sweet potato contains more than 100% of the daily recommended intake. The yellow types contain the most vitamin A. Sweet potatoes are also rich in vitamin B5, vitamin B6, thiamin, niacin, and riboflavin. The orange variety indicates high carotenoid content, while the purple variety is the richest in antioxidants. It also benefits weight loss with its low cholesterol, saturated fatty acid, and salt contents.

PRE-WORKOUT DRINKS

FROZEN CAPPUCCINO

Preparation: 10 minutes   **Servings:** 1

INGREDIENTS

- 1 cup nonfat milk
- ½ cup coffee
- 1 tablespoon cocoa powder
- Ice cubes

PREPARATION

1. Blend all ingredients together.
2. Serve over ice cubes.

NUTRITIONAL INFORMATION

- Calories: 191
- Carbohydrates: 28 grams
- Protein: 13 grams
- Fat: 3 grams

Consumption of two cups of coffee post-workout could reduce muscle pain by 48%. A cup of brewed tea could also boost metabolism by 12%. Caffeine consumption was observed to improve performance by 12%. However, improvement was best after endurance exercise than with shorter periods of training (less than 20 minutes), and was best in athletes who rarely consumed coffee as they were not tolerant to its stimulant effects.

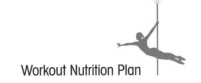

TROPICAL GREEN SMOOTHIE

Preparation: 10 minutes   **Servings:** 1

INGREDIENTS

- ½ cup coconut water
- ½ cup frozen pineapple chunks
- ½ cup frozen mango chunks
- ½ medium banana
- 1 tablespoon frozen spinach

PREPARATION

1. Blend all ingredients together until smooth.
2. Serve immediately or store in the fridge and stir before serving.

NUTRITIONAL INFORMATION

- Calories: 189
- Carbohydrates: 42 grams
- Protein: 3 grams
- Fat: 1 gram

Coconut water is an important treatment for acute diarrhea in some developing countries as it is rich in electrolytes—specifically calcium and magnesium—which may help with stress and muscle tension. Sufficient calcium intake helps keep muscles relaxed—including heart muscles, thus lowering incidents of heart attacks. It also aids with the synthesis of serotonin which elevates mood.

GREEN TEA SMOOTHIE

Preparation: 10 minutes   **Servings:** 1

INGREDIENTS

- ¼ cup strongly brewed green tea
- ½ cup frozen pineapple or oranges
- ½ medium frozen banana
- ½ medium grapefruit
- 1 tablespoon frozen spinach
- 1 teaspoon whey protein of any flavor
- Ice cubes

PREPARATION

1. Blend all ingredients together until smooth.
2. Add ice cubes for a thicker smoothie.

NUTRITIONAL INFORMATION

- Calories: 182
- Carbohydrates: 37.8 grams
- Protein: 5.5 grams
- Fat: 1 gram

Green tea is rich in metabolism-boosting flavonoids called catechins which are excellent sources of antioxidants, thus those consuming green tea lost substantial amount of weight. Using loose leaves rather than tea bags maximizes health benefits obtained from green tea. It is also rich in theanine which helps boost the immune system and prevent infections. Theanine in green tea can help you manage stress and stay relaxed within 40 minutes after drinking green tea as is stimulates the generation of alpha brain waves. In addition, green tea contains polyphenol compounds which block the absorption of cholesterol in the intestines, thus lowering cholesterol levels.

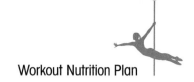

MANGO SMOOTHIE

Preparation: 10 minutes   **Servings:** 1

INGREDIENTS

- ½ cup frozen mango
- ¼ cup coconut water
- ¼ cup nonfat yogurt
- 1 peeled tangerine
- ¼ cup baby carrots
- 2 tablespoon orange juice
- 1 tablespoon frozen spinach

PREPARATION

1. Blend all ingredients together until smooth.

NUTRITIONAL INFORMATION

- Calories: 175
- Carbohydrates: 36 grams
- Protein: 5 grams
- Fat: 1.2 grams

One cup of mango provides about 3 grams of fiber, helping to prevent constipation. They have a sweet, creamy taste, and contain over 20 vitamins and minerals. Mangoes also contribute copper, calcium, and iron to the diet as well as antioxidants such as zeaxanthin and beta-carotene.

CHOCOLATE MINT AVOCADO SMOOTHIE

Preparation: 10 minutes   **Servings:** 1

INGREDIENTS

- ½ cup milk
- ¼ avocado
- 2 teaspoon maple syrup
- 1 tablespoon cocoa powder
- 1 teaspoon peppermint extract
- ½ teaspoon flaxseed
- 1 tablespoon fresh mint
- Ice cubes

PREPARATION

1. Blend ingredients in a mixer without the ice on high speed for 1 minute.

2. Add ice cubes and blend once more on high speed for 30 seconds.

NUTRITIONAL INFORMATION

- Calories: 246
- Carbohydrates: 23 grams
- Protein: 7 grams
- Fat: 14 grams

Avocados—also known as an alligator pear or butter fruit—is the only fruit that provides a substantial amount of healthy monounsaturated fatty acids (MUFA). Avocados contain nearly 20 vitamins and minerals, thus classifying them as a naturally nutrient dense food. Avocados are a great source of vitamins C, E, K, and B6, as well as riboflavin, niacin, folate, pantothenic acid, magnesium, and potassium. They also provide lutein, beta-carotene, and omega-3 fatty acids. They contain substances called saponins which have been associated with relief of symptoms in knee osteoarthritis. It also has antimicrobial defense, particularly against Escherichia coli which is the leading cause of food poisoning.

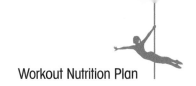

BANANA PEANUT BUTTER SMOOTHIE

Preparation: 10 minutes   **Servings:** 1

INGREDIENTS

- 1 cup nonfat milk
- 1 tablespoon cocoa powder
- 1 tablespoon peanut butter
- ½ cup frozen bananas
- Ice cubes

PREPARATION

1. Blend all ingredients together until smooth.
2. Serve cold.

NUTRITIONAL INFORMATION

- Calories: 295
- Carbohydrates: 40 grams
- Protein: 13.5 grams
- Fat: 9 grams

A serving of peanut butter has 3 mg of vitamin E which is a powerful antioxidant. It is rich in magnesium (49 mg), potassium (208 mg), and immunity-boosting vitamin B6 (0.17 mg). It is also rich in monounsaturated fat which aids in reducing belly fat and has a combination of fiber (2 g per serving) and protein (8 g per serving) that helps keeps you feel full for a longer time.

POST-WORKOUT DRINKS

FIG AND WALNUT YOGURT PARFAIT

Preparation: 5 minutes   **Cooking:** 20 minutes   **Servings:** 1

INGREDIENTS

- 2/3 cup nonfat yogurt
- 2 figs, quartered
- 2 tablespoon walnuts
- 2 tablespoon honey

PREPARATION

1. Preheat oven to 380°F, then place figs and walnuts on a baking sheet to roast for 15 minutes and 8 minutes, respectively. Allow to cool.

2. In a cup, place a layer of yogurt followed by a layer of fig, walnuts, and honey, then repeat.

NUTRITIONAL INFORMATION

- Calories: 348
- Carbohydrates: 50 grams
- Protein: 10 grams
- Fat: 12 grams

Honey has beneficial antibacterial properties; it was used topically to treat cuts and burns even before the discovery of antibiotics. It was also used as a cough suppressant. It consists mainly of sugar and contains a small amount of protein along with small amounts of folate, vitamin C, and other essential vitamins. Yogurt has long been known to improve digestion. The nutritive value and other health benefits increase when honey and yogurt are combined. They can be low in calories when consumed in moderate amounts, thus providing an ideal balance of carbohydrates and proteins. The high glucose content from honey in conjunction with a protein source is an optimal choice for endurance, weight training, and muscle recovery.

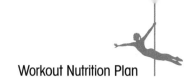

PINEAPPLE PARSLEY SMOOTHIE

Preparation: 10   **Servings:** 1

INGREDIENTS

- ½ cup fresh pineapple
- ½ cup arugula
- ¼ cup fresh parsley
- 1 small cucumber

- ½ medium green apple
- ½ medium grapefruit
- 1 large peeled lemon
- ¼ inch fresh ginger

PREPARATION

1. Blend all ingredients together, then drain.
2. Serve immediately.

NUTRITIONAL INFORMATION

- Calories: 217
- Carbohydrates: 48 grams

- Protein: 4 grams
- Fat: 1 gram

Bromelain is a complex compound that can be extracted from the core of the pineapple which helps reduce severe inflammation and tumor growth. Some studies indicate that bromelain may be helpful in treating osteoarthritis; however, excessive quantities can increase menstrual bleeding and trigger skin rashes as well as vomiting and diarrhea. Pineapple also contains vast amounts of vitamin C, and has the potential to bring about diarrhea, nausea, vomiting, abdominal pain, or heart burn.

POMEGRANATE SMOOTHIE

Preparation: 10 minutes   **Servings:** 1

INGREDIENTS

- ¼ cup low fat yogurt
- ¼ cup pomegranate juice
- ½ cup frozen berries
- ½ cup frozen bananas
- 2 teaspoons honey

PREPARATION

1. Blend all ingredients together until smooth.
2. Serve cold.

NUTRITIONAL INFORMATION

- Calories: 225
- Carbohydrates: 49 grams
- Protein: 5 grams
- Fat: 1 grams

Pomegranate seeds get their vibrant red hue from polyphenols which are powerful antioxidants. Pomegranate juice has three times more antioxidants than red wine and green tea, and contains higher levels of antioxidants than most other fruit juices. It contains 40% of the daily required amounts of vitamin C. For optimal benefits, make pomegranate juice at home as vitamin C breaks down when pasteurized. Pomegranate juice can reduce inflammation in the gut and improve digestion, so it could be beneficial to those with Crohn's disease, ulcerative colitis, or other inflammatory bowel diseases.

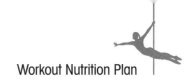

STRAWBERRY OATMEAL SMOOTHIE

Preparation: 10 minutes   **Servings:** 1

INGREDIENTS

- ½ cup nonfat milk
- ½ medium banana
- ¼ cup frozen strawberries
- ¼ cup quick oats
- ¼ teaspoon vanilla extract
- 1 teaspoon honey (optional)

PREPARATION

Blend all ingredients together until smooth.

NUTRITIONAL INFORMATION

- Calories: 214
- Carbohydrates: 41 grams
- Protein: 8 grams
- Fat: 2 grams

Strawberries have powerful anti-inflammatory properties that relieve inflammation and pain associated with several conditions such as the degeneration of muscles, the drying up of joint fluid which affects mobility, or the accumulation of toxic substances and acids as uric acid in the body. It is also rich in vitamin C which stimulates the activity of white blood cells and boosts immunity. Strawberries are rich in iodine and potassium, and are linked to improving cognitive function by regulating brain activity and increasing blood flow.

BERRY SMOOTHIE

Preparation: 15 minutes   **Servings:** 1

INGREDIENTS

- 1 cup skim milk
- 160 g mixed berries
- 1 teaspoon sweetener
- Ice cubes

PREPARATION

Blend all ingredients together until smooth.

NUTRITIONAL INFORMATION

- Calories: 280
- Carbohydrates: 47 g
- Proteins: 12 g
- Fats: 5 g

Berries are rich in antioxidants and polyphenols. They are rich in fiber which promotes digestive health. Having a daily cup of berries for 8 weeks lowers blood pressure and restores HDL (good cholesterol) due to its anthcyanins and ellagic acid.

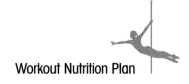

SUN DATE SMOOTHIE

Preparation: 10 minutes   **Servings:** 1

INGREDIENTS

- ½ cup vanilla frozen yogurt
- ¼ cup nonfat milk
- 2 pitted dates, sliced

- 2 tablespoon sun butter
- 5 g whey protein powder of any flavor (optional)

PREPARATION

Blend all ingredients together until smooth.

NUTRITIONAL INFORMATION

- Calories: 431
- Carbohydrates: 42 grams

- Protein: 14 grams
- Fat: 23 grams

Sunflower seeds are rich in vitamin E, calcium, and magnesium. One tablespoon of sunflower seed butter has 24% of the recommended daily intake of vitamin E. Calcium stimulates heart muscles to contract, while magnesium causes them to relax so they synergistically maintain a normal heart rhythm. Magnesium also lowers blood pressure by relaxing the muscles of blood vessel walls.

TURMERIC SMOOTHIE

Preparation: 10 minutes   **Servings:** 1

INGREDIENTS

- ½ cup milk
- ½ cup frozen mango chunks
- ½ a medium banana
- ½ teaspoon coconut oil
- ¼ teaspoon cinnamon
- ¼ teaspoon turmeric powder
- ¼ teaspoon chili

PREPARATION

1. Blend all ingredients together until smooth.
2. Serve immediately.

NUTRITIONAL INFORMATION

- Calories: 194
- Carbohydrates: 33.5 grams
- Protein: 6 grams
- Fat: 4 grams

One of the organic components of turmeric is called curcumin which has antioxidant properties in neural pathways, thus improving cognition. It also boosts immune function. The anti-inflammatory qualities of turmeric decrease joint inflammation and associated pain. The effects of turmeric were found to be comparable with pharmaceutical products such as ibuprofen.

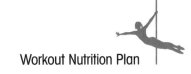

POST-WORKOUT SNACKS

PITA NACHOS AND CRAB DIP

Preparation: 15 minutes   **Cooking:** 15 minutes   **Servings:** 1

INGREDIENTS

For the pita nachos:

- 1 small pita bread, quartered
- ½ tablespoon olive oil

For the crab dip:

- 1.5 ounce crab meat
- 1 tablespoon sour cream
- 1 tablespoon mayonnaise
- ½ tablespoon chopped scallions
- 1/8 celery stick, chopped
- 1 teaspoon olive oil
- 1 teaspoon lemon juice
- 1 teaspoon chopped fresh parsley
- 1 teaspoon chopped fresh chives
- ½ teaspoon white pepper
- ½ teaspoon black pepper
- ¼ teaspoon salt

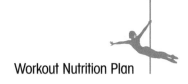

PREPARATION

For the pita nachos:

1. Spread pita sections on a baking sheet and drizzle with olive oil.

2. Bake at 300 °F for 5 minutes per side.

For the crab dip:

1. Mix all ingredients—except for the celery and chives—together.

2. Serve with celery and chives on top.

Nutritional information

- Calories: 383
- Carbohydrates: 24 grams
- Protein: 11 grams
- Fat: 27 grams

Pita bread has 5.5 grams of protein, 33 grams of carbohydrates, and 1 gram of fiber. Whole-wheat pita bread, on the other hand, has more than 6 grams of fiber per serving as well as higher levels of magnesium and vitamin B. White pita is also high in selenium which is over 30% of the recommended intake and has 322 milligrams of salt in one serving despite not being salty.

WATERMELON AND CHEESE

Preparation: 10 minutes   **Servings:** 1

INGREDIENTS

- 2 slices (4 oz) of watermelon, cubed
- 2 ounces cottage cheese
- 2 ounces blueberries
- ½ cup watercress

PREPARATION

Serve with cottage cheese, blueberries, and watercress.

NUTRITIONAL INFORMATION

- Calories: 153
- Carbohydrates: 20 grams
- Protein: 11.3 grams
- Fat: 3

Watercress contains more vitamin C than an orange, more calcium than milk, more iron than spinach, and more folate than bananas. Folate levels protect against the deterioration of cognitive functions and the risk of depression. Its levels could be affected by alcohol consumption.

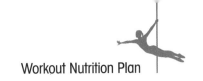

MELON PLUM SALAD

Preparation: 10 minutes **Servings:** 1

INGREDIENTS

- 1 cup watermelon, seeded and cubed
- 1 cup honeydew melon balls
- 2 small red plums, sliced
- ½ cup watercress, torn
- ¼ cup feta cheese, crumbled
- 1 teaspoon sweet chili sauce
- ½ teaspoon salt

PREPARATION

1. Mix all ingredients—except sweet chili sauce and salt—in a bowl.

2. Season with sweet chili sauce and salt, then serve immediately.

NUTRITIONAL INFORMATION

- Calories: 332
- Carbohydrates: 53 grams
- Protein: 9 grams
- Fat: 9.3 grams

Watermelons are rich in fiber and citrulline. Citrulline is an amino acid that converts to arginine in the body which in turn improves blood flow and cardiovascular health. The white flesh nearest the rind has even higher levels of citrulline. Watermelons are also rich in lycopene which yields high anti-inflammatory and antioxidant properties. Drinking watermelon juice before an intense workout helps to reduce soreness the following day. However, consumption of more than 30 mg of lycopene per day could potentially cause nausea, diarrhea, bloating, and indigestion, thus watermelon should be consumed in moderation.

RED BELL PEPPERS, ORANGES, AND YOGURT

Preparation: 10 minutes **Servings:** 1

INGREDIENTS

- 1 medium red bell pepper, julienned
- 1 medium orange, cut into quarters
- 2/3 cup skim yogurt

PREPARATION

Serve bell pepper and orange with yogurt.

NUTRITIONAL INFORMATION

- Calories: 189
- Carbohydrates: 33 grams
- Proteins: 9 grams
- Fats: 2.3 grams

This recipe is very light and rich in vitamin C which boosts post-workout immunity. Red peppers contain capsaicin which is a powerful anti-inflammatory and brings relief from pain.

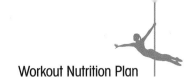

CHERRY TOMATOES AND CHEESE

Preparation: 10 minutes   **Servings:** 1

INGREDIENTS

- 3 cup (150 g) cherry tomatoes, halved
- 15 g cottage cheese
- 15 g goat cheese
- 1 small bunch watercress

PREPARATION

Serve cherry tomato halves with cheese and watercress.

NUTRITIONAL INFORMATION

- Calories: 165
- Carbohydrates: 19 grams
- Protein: 11 grams
- Fat: 5

Goat cheese has 5 grams of protein and 40 mg calcium, along with about 3% of your daily iron requirements. Goat milk, compared to cow milk, increases absorption of iron and improves bone formation and the bioavailability of certain minerals.

HARDBOILED EGG AND CHICKPEA DIP

Preparation: 10 minutes   **Cooking:** 20 minutes   **Servings:** 1

INGREDIENTS

- 1 egg
- 100 grams canned chickpeas
- 1 garlic clove, chopped
- 2 tablespoon olive oil
- 2 tablespoon lemon juice
- 3 tablespoon warm water
- ½ teaspoon chili powder
- Dash of salt and pepper

PREPARATION

1. Boil the egg for 15 to 20 minutes.
2. Combine all ingredients in a food processor and blend until smooth.
3. Drizzle some olive oil and chili over top for serving.

NUTRITIONAL INFORMATION

- Calories: 381
- Carbohydrates: 4 grams
- Protein: 8 grams
- Fat: 37 grams

Chickpeas are also called garbanzo beans. Chickpeas are high in both protein and fiber. They have fat-burning properties and induce satiety which aids and sustains weight loss. Chickpeas are even more filling if paired with other nutritious whole foods.

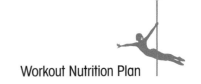

SARDINES AND CRACKERS

Preparation: 5 minutes   **Servings:** 1

INGREDIENTS

- 1 ounce canned sardines
- 4 unsalted crackers
- 1 tablespoon hot sauce

PREPARATION

1. Rinse and drain the sardines to wash off excess salt.
2. Serve with unsalted crackers and hot sauce.

NUTRITIONAL INFORMATION

- Calories: 192
- Carbohydrates: 10 grams
- Protein: 13.2 grams
- Fat: 11 grams

Sardines are one of the richest sources of essential omega-3 fatty acids. Three ounces of sardines provide 338% vitamin B12, 87% selenium, 64% phosphorus, 61% omega-3 fats, 44% vitamin D, 35% calcium, 30% vitamin B3, 24% iodine, 19% copper, and 16% choline.

BLUEBERRY AND PEACH QUINOA CRUMBLE

Preparation: 15 minutes   Cooking: 50 minutes   Servings: 12

INGREDIENTS

For the fruit filling:

- 240 grams blueberries
- 240 grams peaches, peeled and sliced
- 2 tablespoons corn starch
- 2 tablespoons brown sugar

For the crumble:

- 1 cup flour
- ¼ cup rolled oats
- ½ cup cooked quinoa
- ¼ cup brown sugar
- ½ teaspoon salt
- ½ teaspoon cinnamon

PREPARATION

For the fruit filling:

1. Combine peaches and blueberries with corn starch and brown sugar
2. Grease a pan using cooking spray or coconut oil, then pour the mixture into the pan.

For the crumble:

1. In another bowl, mix flour, cooked quinoa, oats, brown sugar, salt, cinnamon, and coconut oil until moist and crumbly.
2. Cover the fruit filling with the crumble.
3. Preheat the oven to 350 °F and bake for 50 minutes.

NUTRITIONAL INFORMATION

Each serving (60 grams)

- Calories: 107
- Carbohydrates: 23.7 grams
- Proteins: 2 grams
- Fats: 0.4 grams

Peaches are rich in potassium and vitamin C, so they reduce muscle cramps. They are also rich in magnesium, providing a calming effect to the nervous system. They are good detoxifiers, and they keep bad cholesterol low. They are good sources of calcium for vegans.

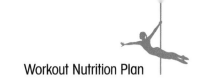

HONEY ALMOND OAT BALLS

Preparation: 90 minutes   **Servings:** 12

INGREDIENTS

- 2 cups quick oats
- 1 cup whole roasted nuts, chopped
- ½ cup dried fruits (dried apricots, prunes, dates, and different types of raisins)
- ½ cup honey
- 2/3 cup almond butter

PREPARATION

1. In one bowl, combine oats, dried fruits, and chopped nuts. In another bowl, combine honey and almond butter, then add to oat mixture.

2. Line an 8 x 8 pan with parchment paper and press the mixture into the pan with damp hands.

3. Cover with plastic wrap and refrigerate for 2 hours.

4. Cut into 12 pieces and form into balls with damp hands, then serve.

NUTRITIONAL INFORMATION

Each serving (30 grams)

- Calories: 243
- Carbohydrates: 30 grams
- Protein: 6 grams
- Fat: 11 grams

Wild almonds or bitter almonds contain glycoside amygdalin. Once an almond is crushed or chewed, it is converted to prussic acid (hydrogen cyanide) which is a deadly poison, but sweet almonds do not contain glycoside amygdale. Almonds are a good source of vitamin E, copper, and magnesium. They also contain high levels of healthy unsaturated fatty acids and bioactive compounds. Nuts and seeds are rich in fiber and therefore are of benefit to cardiovascular health.

APPLE OATMEAL SNACK BARS

Preparation: 20 minutes   **Cooking:** 30 minutes   **Servings:** 12

INGREDIENTS

For the oatmeal bars:

- 1 cup flour
- 1 ½ cup rolled oats
- 2 tablespoons brown sugar
- 1 teaspoon cinnamon
- ¼ teaspoon salt
- ¼ teaspoon baking soda
- Pinch nutmeg

For the apple filling:

- 1 medium apple, chopped
- ½ cup unsweetened applesauce
- ½ cup apple butter
- ¼ cup coconut oil
- ¼ cup maple syrup

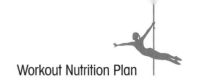

PREPARATION

1. Preheat oven to 320 ˚F, then grease an 8 x 8 pan with coconut oil.

2. In a bowl, mix oats, flour, sugar, cinnamon, nutmeg, and baking soda.

3. In another bowl, mix chopped apples, applesauce, apple butter, maple syrup, and coconut oil.

4. Press half of the oat mixture into the pan, then top with the apple mixture.

5. Place the rest of the oat mixture over the layer of apple mixture.

6. Bake for 30 minutes.

7. Allow it to cool, then cut into 12 bars.

8. Bars may be stored in the refrigerator for up to 10 days.

NUTRITIONAL INFORMATION

Each serving (50 grams)

- Calories: 185
- Carbohydrates: 32 grams
- Protein: 3 grams
- Fat: 5 grams

Apples are rich in vitamin C, vitamin B complex, polyphenol compounds with powerful antioxidant activity, and minerals such as calcium (6 mg), magnesium (5 mg), potassium (107 mg), and phosphorous (11 mg). However, apples are also fairly acidic, and could be up to four times more damaging to the teeth than carbonated drinks. Eating acidic foods at meal times is much healthier than snacking on apples throughout the day.

COCONUT RICE PUDDING

Preparation: 10 minutes · **Cooking:** 30 minutes · **Servings:** 1

INGREDIENTS

- 1/8 cup medium-grain rice
- ½ cup water
- ¼ cup whole milk
- ¼ cup coconut milk
- 2 teaspoon caster sugar (or powdered sugar)
- ¼ teaspoon vanilla extract
- Coconut flakes, crushed nuts, or sliced fruits for serving

PREPARATION

1. In a small saucepan, mix rice, milk, sugar, vanilla, and water.
2. Bring mixture to a boil, then lower the heat and simmer for 15 to 25 minutes.
3. Serve with your choice of nuts, fruits, or coconut flakes.

NUTRITIONAL INFORMATION

- Calories: 318
- Carbohydrates: 37 grams
- Protein: 5 grams
- Fat: 16.6 grams

Unlike cow milk, coconut milk is lactose free. It is a good choice for vegans. Coconuts are highly nutritious and rich in fiber, vitamin C, vitamin E, vitamin B complex, and minerals as iron, selenium, sodium, calcium, phosphorous, and magnesium.

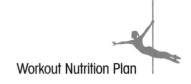

TERESITA'S LECHE FLAN

Preparation: 150 minutes   **Cooking:** 30 minutes   **Servings:** 1

INGREDIENTS

- 1 whole egg
- 1 egg yolk
- 1 cup whole milk
- 2 tablespoon sugar
- Dash of vanilla extract

PREPARATION

1. Add 1½ tablespoon sugar to the milk.

2. Bring milk to a boil, then set it aside to cool down.

3. Whisk eggs, then add to the milk.

4. In a small pan, add the remaining sugar and a few drops of water.

5. Pour the milk mixture into the pan.

6. Place some water in a pot and bring it to a boil.

7. Place a colander over the pot, and place the small pan with the milk mixture into the colander. Cover with a lid.

8. Steam the flan for 20 minutes or until a toothpick comes out clean.

9. Refrigerate for 2 hours before serving.

NUTRITIONAL INFORMATION

- Calories: 446
- Carbohydrates: 37 grams
- Protein: 20.5 grams
- Fat: 24 grams

Cow milk is a rich source of essential proteins. Whole milk is also a rich source of saturated fat which is used as an alternative source of energy and which preserves muscle mass (maintaining lean muscle mass is essential for weight management). Milk is also a rich source of choline which is an important nutrient found to support sleep and muscle movement. Dairy proteins can support muscle growth and repair.

POST-WORKOUT MEALS

BLACK BEAN AVOCADO SALAD

Preparation: 15 minutes   **Servings:** 1

INGREDIENTS

- ¼ avocado, chopped
- 2 ounces black beans
- 2 ounces frozen sweet corn
- 1 tablespoon chopped onions
- 1 tablespoon sliced medium tomato
- 1 tablespoon diced red bell peppers
- 2 tablespoon chopped cilantro
- 2 tablespoon lime juice
- 1 tablespoon olive oil
- Dash salt and pepper

PREPARATION

1. Mix all ingredients together.
2. Refrigerate for 30 minutes.
3. Serve chilled.

NUTRITIONAL INFORMATION

- Calories: 494
- Carbohydrates: 58 grams
- Protein: 16 grams
- Fat: 22 grams

This recipe is a good choice for gluten-intolerant individuals. Sweet corn is gluten free. Despite being sweet, 63 grams of sweet corn has nearly same amount of calories as an apple and has a lower sugar content. It is rich in fiber—2.7 grams per 100 grams—specifically insoluble fibers, which are very good for gut health. It is loaded with phytochemicals such as lutein and zeaxanthin which protect your retina against oxidative damage, and its antioxidant activity increases with cooking.

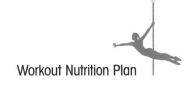

COWPEA SALAD

Preparation: 15 minutes   **Cooking:** 20 minutes   **Servings:** 1

INGREDIENTS

- 2 ounces cowpeas
- 2 tablespoon diced red bell pepper
- 2 tablespoon diced fresh parsley
- 1 tablespoon sliced yellow onions
- 1 tablespoon quinoa
- 1 teaspoon diced chili pepper
- 1 teaspoon vegetable oil
- 1 tablespoon lemon juice
- 1 tablespoon olive oil
- ½ teaspoon black pepper

PREPARATION

1. Place cowpeas in water and bring to a boil over medium heat. Lower heat and simmer for 20 minutes or until tender.

2. Simmer quinoa for 3 minutes.

3. Sauté onion slices with minced garlic and vegetable oil.

4. Combine cowpeas, quinoa, and sautéed onions, then add red bell peppers, chili, and parsley.

5. Season with olive oil, lemon juice, and black pepper.

NUTRITIONAL INFORMATION

- Calories: 353
- Carbohydrates: 33 grams
- Protein: 8 grams
- Fat: 21 grams

Cowpeas have high levels of tryptophan which can help the body relax and sleep. They are rich in magnesium which plays an important role in the metabolism of carbohydrates and can help the body maintain balanced levels of blood sugar. These beans are very low in calories and cholesterol, which benefits weight loss. Their high fiber content promotes better digestion.

TUNA SANDWICH

Preparation: 15 minutes   **Servings:** 1

INGREDIENTS

- 1 ounce tuna
- 1 teaspoon diced celery stalk
- 1 teaspoon diced spring onion
- 1 tablespoon light mayonnaise
- ½ tsp lemon juice
- Dash of salt
- Dash of pepper
- 2 white toasts

PREPARATION

1. Drain the tuna.
2. Mix all ingredients.
3. Spread over white toasts.

NUTRITIONAL INFORMATION

- Calories: 356
- Carbohydrates: 35.4 grams
- Proteins: 13 grams
- Fats: 18 grams

Tuna is a good choice for pescetarians—especially after endurance activities—as it is packed with proteins and iron. It is rich in omega-3 fatty acids which stimulate the leptin hormone and induce satiety, bringing back your appetite balance. It is rich in vitamin B complex which benefits and boosts metabolism. It is also rich in zinc, manganese, and vitamin C, and contains nearly 200% of the daily requirements of selenium, making it a powerful antioxidant and guarding against inflammations.

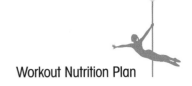

SHRIMP SALAD

Preparation: 90 minutes   **Cooking:** 10 minutes   **Servings:** 1

INGREDIENTS

- 3 ounces shrimp
- 1 tablespoon chopped fresh parsley
- 1 tablespoon mayonnaise
- ½ tablespoon diced red onions
- ½ tablespoon orange juice

- ½ tablespoon lemon juice
- 1 teaspoon orange zest
- 1 teaspoon olive oil
- 1 teaspoon vinegar
- Dash of salt and pepper

PREPARATION

1. Preheat oven to 400 °F, then place shrimp on a baking sheet and toss with olive oil and a dash of salt and pepper. Bake for 7 minutes.

2. In a small bowl, whisk mayonnaise, lemon juice, orange juice, and orange zest, then add red onions and parsley.

3. Fold the shrimps into the sauce and chill for 1 hour.

4. Serve at room temperature.

NUTRITIONAL INFORMATION

- Calories: 252
- Carbohydrates: 5.5 grams

- Protein: 18 grams
- Fat: 17.5 grams

There are around 8.2 mg of vitamin C in 1 tablespoon of orange zest. It greatly benefits gut health by relieving constipation due its insoluble fibers. Orange zest contains a huge variety of flavonoids and phytonutrients, so it is recommended to sprinkle a little over salads, vegetables, or even desserts.

TUNA PASTA SALAD

Preparation: 10 minutes   **Cooking:** 15 minutes   **Servings:** 1

INGREDIENTS

- 2 ounce tuna
- 2 ounce pasta
- 2 tablespoon diced tomato
- 2 tablespoon diced celery stalk
- 1 tablespoon mayonnaise

- 1 teaspoon lemon juice
- 1 teaspoon honey
- 1 teaspoon black pepper
- 1 teaspoon vegetable oil
- Dash of salt

PREPARATION

1. In a saucepan, boil pasta in a pot of salted water until tender, then rinse in cold water and drain.

2. Prepare dressing by whisking together the mayonnaise, lemon juice, and honey, then add tomatoes and celery.

3. Combine the tuna with the pasta and dressing.

NUTRITIONAL INFORMATION

- Calories: 577
- Carbohydrates: 56 grams

- Protein: 23 grams
- Fat: 29 grams

Celery is low in calories and contains vital nutrients which regulate fat metabolism. It also provides antioxidants which help improve liver function and benefit weight loss. It has a high water and electrolyte content which helps prevent dehydration. It has also been used as an antihypertensive agent for centuries due to its diuretic effect. Celery protects against stomach ulcers due to its ethanol extract which replenishes the mucus lining of the stomach

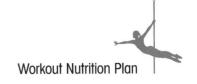

LEMON SALMON STEAK

Preparation: 10 minutes   **Cooking:** 25 minutes   **Servings:** 1

INGREDIENTS

- 3 ounce salmon steak
- 2 ounce water
- 1 medium tomato, chopped
- ½ cup fresh cilantro, chopped
- 1 tablespoon olive oil

- ½ tablespoon butter
- ½ teaspoon minced garlic
- 1 tablespoon lemon juice
- Dash of salt and pepper

PREPARATION

1. Over medium heat, heat the oil and butter in a small skillet, then add the minced garlic and sauté for 1 minute.

2. Place the salmon in the skillet and season with lemon juice, salt, and pepper.

3. Add the chopped tomatoes and the fresh cilantro and sauté for another minute.

4. Add the water, then cover the skillet for 10 to 15 minutes.

NUTRITIONAL INFORMATION

- Calories: 393
- Carbohydrates: 4 grams

- Protein: 20 grams
- Fat: 33 grams

Salmon is a fatty fish very rich in omega-3 fatty acids and vitamin B complex which aids the metabolic processes. It is also rich in vitamin D and selenium which, together with omega-3 fatty acids, improve brain function. This also can benefit children by improving their memory and their academic performance and protecting against ADHD symptoms. Selenium has antioxidant properties which is very beneficial for workouts.

MEATLOAF AND TABBOULEH

Preparation: 30 minutes   **Cooking:** 75 minutes   **Servings:** 1

INGREDIENTS

For the meatloaf (12 servings):

- 750 g ground beef
- 2 tablespoon bread crumbs
- 1 egg
- 1 small red onion

- 1 teaspoon salt
- ½ teaspoon black pepper
- 4 tablespoon ketchup
- ½ cup semi-skim milk

For the meat sauce:

- 4 Tablespoon apple cider vinegar
- 2 Tablespoon dark brown sugar

- ½ cup ketchup

For the tabbouleh (one serving):

- 1 tablespoon quinoa
- 1 tablespoon olive oil
- 1 tablespoon lemon
- 1 cup parsley, chopped
- ¼ cup fresh mint leaves, chopped

- 1 tablespoon diced tomato
- 1 tablespoon sliced cucumber
- ¼ teaspoon salt
- ¼ teaspoon black pepper

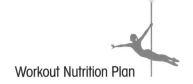

PREPARATION

For the meatloaf:

1. Combine meatloaf ingredients and spread in a loaf pan.

2. Combine meat sauce ingredients in a separate bowl.

3. Pour the sauce over the meatloaf.

4. Bake at 350˚ F for 60-90 minutes, until done.

For the tabbouleh:

1. In a small saucepan, boil quinoa for 3 minutes. Set aside to cool, then drain.

2. In a small bowl, mix mint, parsley, tomato, cucumber, and a squeeze of lemon juice.

3. Add quinoa, salt, and black pepper.

NUTRITIONAL INFORMATION

One serving of meatloaf (one slice)

- Calories: 187
- Carbohydrates: 9 grams

- Protein: 13 grams
- Fat: 11 grams

Tabbouleh

- Calories: 204
- Carbohydrates: 11 grams

- Protein: 4 grams
- Fat: 16 grams

Myricetin is a flavonoid found in parsley which has been shown to reduce incidence of skin cancer, so it is recommended to pair green vegetables with charred grilled food, which has been linked to several types of cancer.

BRUSSELS SPROUTS AND GRILLED BURGER

Preparation: 25 minutes   **Cooking:** 20 minutes   **Servings:** 1

INGREDIENTS

For the grilled burger:

- 1 pound minced meat
- Dash of salt and pepper

For the Brussels sprouts

- 2 ounces Brussels sprouts, shredded
- ¼ avocado, diced
- ½ clementine, peeled and sliced
- 1 tablespoon grapefruit
- 1 tablespoon extra virgin olive oil

- 1 teaspoon Dijon mustard

- 1 teaspoon minced garlic
- 1 teaspoon black pepper
- ¼ teaspoon salt
- ¼ cup pistachios (optional)

PREPARATION

For the grilled burger:

1. Shape minced meat into 2 balls; then flatten.

2. Sprinkle salt and pepper on both sides.

3. Heat the pan for 5 minutes.

4. Brush both sides of the burger with vegetable oil.

5. Grill each side for 10 minutes.

6. Brush both sides with mustard.

7. Grill each side for another 10 minutes, and then serve.

For the Brussels sprouts:

1. Mix Brussels sprouts, clementine, avocado, and pistachios (if using).

2. Prepare dressing by combining olive oil, grapefruit juice, garlic, salt, and pepper.

3. Toss in Brussels sprouts, clementine, avocado, and pistachio mixture.

4. Chill, then serve.

NUTRITIONAL INFORMATION

Without pistachios
- Calories: 419
- Carbohydrates: 16 grams
- Protein: 19 grams
- Fat: 31 grams

With pistachios
- Calories: 536
- Carbohydrates: 16 grams
- Protein: 19 grams
- Fat: 44 grams

Brussels sprouts are high in protein. One serving provides the daily requirements of vitamin C and vitamin K which means that caution should be considered when on blood-thinning medications. Many green vegetables contain α-lipoic acid which has antioxidant properties, lowers blood glucose levels, and increases insulin sensitivity. Brussels sprouts provide 75 mg of α-lipoic acid per cup which is over 100% of the daily requirements. Oven-roasting Brussels sprouts brings out their sweet taste and keeps them crispy while diminishing their sulfurous taste. Overcooking can reduce mineral content.

WHITE FISH WITH TOMATO AND PARSLEY

Preparation: 30 minutes   **Cooking:** 15 minutes   **Servings:** 1

INGREDIENTS

For the white fish:

- 3 ounces white fish (any type)
- 1 garlic clove, minced
- ¼ teaspoon dried rosemary
- 2 tablespoon fresh parsley
- 1 tablespoon lemon juice

- 1 tablespoon olive oil
- ¼ teaspoon salt
- ¼ teaspoon white pepper
- ¼ teaspoon black pepper

For the tomato and parsley:

- 1 medium tomato, de-seeded and diced
- 1 tablespoon diced red onion

- 1 tablespoon chopped fresh parsley
- Dash of salt and pepper

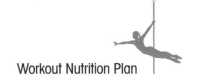

PREPARATION

For the white fish:

1. Mix olive oil with minced garlic, dried rosemary, fresh parsley, lemon juice, salt, and pepper.

2. Use mixture to coat white fish.

3. Wrap white fish in foil and top with any remaining mixture.

4. Place wrapped fish in a baking tin. Bake at 325° F for 15 minutes.

Tomato and parsley

1. Combine ingredients and season with salt and pepper.

NUTRITIONAL INFORMATION

- Calories: 347
- Carbohydrates: 11 grams
- Protein: 24 grams
- Fat: 23 grams

In addition to vitamin E and vitamin C, tomatoes also contain four types of antioxidants: alpha-carotene, beta-carotene, lutein, and lycopene which make them very rich in antioxidant activity. Ingestion of healthy fats increases lycopene absorption up to 15 times.

Dried rosemary is a good source of calcium, iron, vitamin C, and vitamin B6. Based on a 2,000-calorie diet, it provides 55% of the daily recommended amount of magnesium, 62% of vitamin A, 102% of vitamin C, 128% of calcium, 162% of iron, and 85 % of vitamin B6.

CHICKEN PASTA

Preparation: 15 minutes   **Cooking:** 20 minutes   **Servings:** 1

INGREDIENTS

- 3 ounce chicken
- 2 ounce pasta
- 1 ounce sliced artichoke
- 1 tablespoon sliced tomatoes
- 1 tablespoon sliced red onion
- ½ teaspoon minced garlic
- 1 tablespoon olive oil
- 1 teaspoon vegetable oil
- 1 tablespoon fresh parsley
- ½ tablespoon lemon juice
- ½ teaspoon oregano
- 1 ounce crumbled feta cheese

PREPARATION

1. Boil the pasta in a pot of salted water, then rinse with cold water and drain.

2. Steam the artichoke.

3. In another pan over medium heat, heat oil with onion and garlic, and add chicken. Cook until chicken is tender.

4. Combine pasta, chicken, artichoke, and sliced tomatoes.

5. Prepare seasoning by combining olive oil, lemon juice, oregano, salt, and pepper. Add to the salad.

6. Garnish with feta cheese and parsley.

NUTRITIONAL INFORMATION

- Calories: 326
- Carbohydrates: 31 grams
- Protein: 28 grams
- Fat: 10 grams

Cynarin is a compound found in artichokes which increases bile production, helps speed up food movement through the intestine, and reduces bloating. Inulin is another fiber found in artichokes which acts as a prebiotic, aiding probiotics in the gut. The phytonutrients in artichokes also provide more antioxidants in one serving than even dark chocolate, blueberries, or red wine. There is a wide range of antioxidants that boost immunity and improve cardiovascular health.

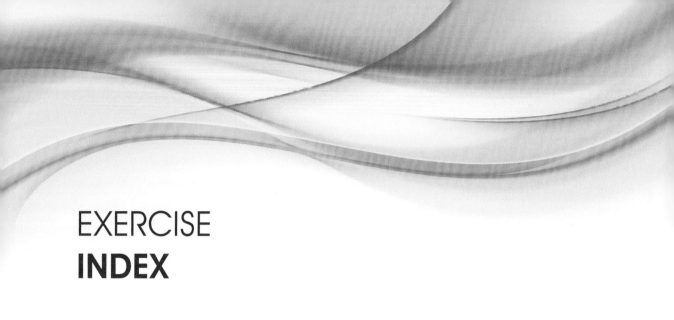

EXERCISE
INDEX

CHAPTER 1 POSITIONS AND POLE PRINCIPLES

BODY POSITION

HAND GRIPS AND ARM POSITIONS

LEG POSITIONS

CHAPTER 2 PRE-WORKOUT STRETCHING

UPPER-BODY MOBILITY AND STRETCH EXERCISES

LOWER-BODY MOBILITY STRETCH EXERCISES

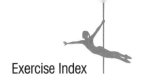

CHAPTER 3 WARM-UPS

INDIVIDUAL WORKOUTS

POLE WORKOUTS

CHAPTER 4 POLE POSTURAL EXERCISES

POSTURAL EXERCISES

CHAPTER 5 TRANSITIONAL MOVEMENTS

TRANSITIONAL MOVEMENTS

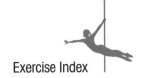

CHAPTER 6 CLIMBS

CLIMBS

CHAPTER 7 SHOULDER MOUNTS

SHOULDER MOUNTS

CHAPTER 8 HANDSTANDS

HANDSTANDS

CHAPTER 9 POLE DANCE PROGRAM

BASIC

POLE DANCE FITNESS

- Pole hug fang (embrace) 211
- Pencil spin baseball grip 211
- Pole hug (one-arm embrace) 211
- Scissor spin baseball grip 212
- Super girl 212
- Rocket man 212
- Yogini 213
- Twisted yogini 213
- Armpit hold straddle (teddy) 213
- Armpit hold (teddy variation) 214
- Layback (crossed knee) 214
- Basic rainbow 214
- Closed crossed knee release 215
- Stargazer 215
- Liberty 215
- Shishi spin 216
- Layback crossed ankle 216
- Pixie 217
- Crescent moon 217
- Bow and arrow 218
- Inverted pencil 218
- Iguana fang 219

INTERMEDIATE

- Inverted pencil V 222
- Cupid supported 222
- Dart 223
- Tuck drop 223
- Spaceflight 223
- Side V 224
- Inversion leg hold 224
- Inversion legs tucked 225
- Inverted crucifix 225
- Inversion legs extended 225
- Horizontal dismount 226
- Pencil full bracket split grip 226
- Air walk 226
- Basic inverted split 227
- Gemini attitude 227
- Top-handed outside knee hook 228
- Scorpion 228
- Scorpion attitude 228
- Scorpion hold (dragon) 229
- Scorpion flatliner 229
- Scorpion (foot hold) 229
- Static electric leg switch 230
- Cocoon 230
- Bow and arrow (one hand) 231
- Jasmine 231
- Dragonfly (Inverted thigh hold) 232
- Side pole straddle 232
- Dragonfly crossed 232

ADVANCED

CHAPTER 11 POST WORKOUT STRETCHING

POST WORKOUT STRETCHES

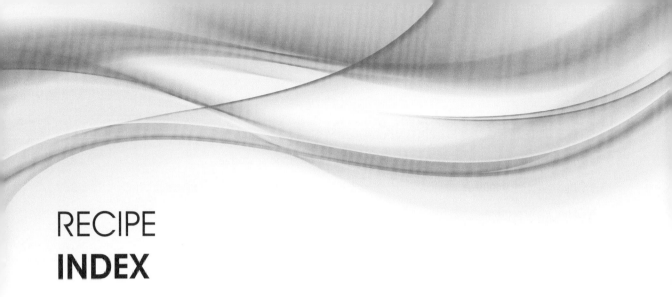

RECIPE
INDEX

PRE-WORKOUT MEALS

PRE-WORKOUT SNACKS

PRE-WORKOUT DRINKS

POST-WORKOUT DRINKS

POST-WORKOUT SNACKS

POST-WORKOUT MEALS